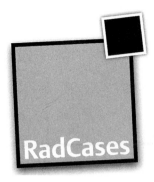

# Neuro Imaging

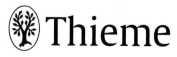

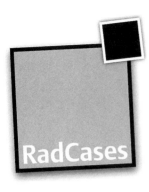

# Neuro Imaging

Edited by

**Roy Riascos, MD**
Associate Professor of Radiology
Department of Radiology
The University of Texas Medical Branch
Galveston, Texas

**Eliana Bonfante, MD**
Assistant Professor
Department of Diagnostic and Interventional Imaging
University of Texas Medical School at Houston
Houston, Texas


Series Editors
**Jonathan Lorenz, MD**
Associate Professor of Radiology
Department of Radiology
The University of Chicago
Chicago, Illinois

**Hector Ferral, MD**
Professor of Radiology
Section Chief, Interventional Radiology
RUSH University Medical Center, Chicago
Chicago, Illinois

Thieme
New York • Stuttgart

Thieme Medical Publishers, Inc.
333 Seventh Ave.
New York, NY 10001

Executive Editor: Timothy Hiscock
Editorial Assistant: Adriana di Giorgio
Editorial Director: Michael Wachinger
Production Editor: Katy Whipple, Maryland Composition
International Production Director: Andreas Schabert
Vice President, International Marketing and Sales: Cornelia Schulze
Chief Financial Officer: James W. Mitos
President: Brian D. Scanlan
Compositor: MPS Content Services
Printer: Sheridan Press

Library of Congress Cataloging-in-Publication Data

Neuro imaging / edited by Roy F. Riascos and Eliana E. Bonfante.
     p. ; cm. — (RadCases)
  Includes bibliographical references.
  Summary: This book is not intended to teach neuroradiology—it is only a review of the most frequent pathologies and serves as a tool to be able to tell them apart. Of course, telling them apart is not always possible, and
that is the whole trick of giving a pertinent set of differential diagnoses and trying to favor one over the other.
Our advice is to always look at the first image and try to describe as much as you can, as if it was the only image
you had available, then go through the rest of the images and see if the thought process was similar. It would be
impossible to include all the pertinent differential diagnoses for each case with the format limitation of three
differential diagnoses per case. This way of teaching imaging analysis can both be similar to and very different
from your daily clinical practice. Often, the pertinent finding or telltale sign to achieve a diagnosis lies in just a
few of the images within an entire examination; however, you have to see the entire case and find these. Here,
images that have been deemed key by someone else are selected, giving you the advantage of a focused search
but the limitation of a narrow representation. You may find yourself frustrated by offering a totally different
differential diagnosis from the one presented to you here, but be aware that the same case can have a completely different approach based on the way it is presented, the order of the images, or the finding in which you
are focusing your process of thought. Additional references are provided to help you widen the scope of your
review, especially in subjects that you may find more challenging or controversial—Provided by publisher.
  ISBN 978-1-60406-189-5
  1. Nervous system—Radiography—Case studies. I. Riascos, Roy F. II. Bonfante, Eliana E. III. Series: RadCases.
  [DNLM: 1. Central Nervous System Diseases—radiography—Case Reports. 2. Central Nervous System—
radiography—Case Reports. 3. Diagnostic Techniques, Neurological—Case Reports. WL 141 N4825 2010]
  RC349.R3N33 2010
  616.8'047572—dc22
                                                                                             2010020830

**Important note:** Medical knowledge is ever-changing. As new research and clinical experience broaden our
knowledge, changes in treatment and drug therapy may be required. The authors and editors of the material
herein have consulted sources believed to be reliable in their efforts to provide information that is complete
and in accord with the standards accepted at the time of publication. However, in view of the possibility of
human error by the authors, editors, or publisher of the work herein or changes in medical knowledge, nei-
ther the authors, editors, nor publisher, nor any other party who has been involved in the preparation of this
work, warrants that the information contained herein is in every respect accurate or complete, and they are
not responsible for any errors or omissions or for the results obtained from use of such information. Readers
are encouraged to confirm the information contained herein with other sources. For example, readers are
advised to check the product information sheet included in the package of each drug they plan to administer
to be certain that the information contained in this publication is accurate and that changes have not been
made in the recommended dose or in the contraindications for administration. This recommendation is of
particular importance in connection with new or infrequently used drugs.

Some of the product names, patents, and registered designs referred to in this book are in fact registered
trademarks or proprietary names even though specific reference to this fact is not always made in the text.
Therefore, the appearance of a name without designation as proprietary is not to be construed as a representation by the publisher that it is in the public domain.

Printed in the United States

978-1-60406-189-5

To the woman for whom my heart surrenders, Maria Claudia, and our three sons,
Camilo, Felipe, and Pablo, for making my life this wonderful experience.
—*Roy Riascos*

This book is dedicated to my loving and supporting soulmate, Darren,
and to our two wonderful and inspiring children, Matthew and Zachary.
—*Eliana Bonfante*

# RadCases Series Preface

The ability to assimilate detailed information across the entire spectrum of radiology is the Holy Grail sought by those preparing for the American Board of Radiology examination. As enthusiastic partners in the Thieme RadCases Series who formerly took the examination, we understand the exhaustion and frustration shared by residents and the families of residents engaged in this quest. It has been our observation that despite ongoing efforts to improve Web-based interactive databases, residents still find themselves searching for material they can review while preparing for the radiology board examinations and remain frustrated by the fact that only a few printed guidebooks are available, which are limited in both format and image quality. Perhaps their greatest source of frustration is the inability to easily locate groups of cases across all subspecialties of radiology that are organized and tailored for their immediate study needs. Imagine being able to immediately access groups of high-quality cases to arrange study sessions, quickly extract and master information, and prepare for theme-based radiology conferences. Our goal in creating the RadCases Series was to combine the popularity and portability of printed books with the adaptability, exceptional quality, and interactive features of an electronic case-based format.

The intent of the printed book is to encourage repeated priming in the use of critical information by providing a portable group of exceptional core cases that the resident can master. The best way to determine the format for these cases was to ask residents from around the country to weigh in. Overwhelmingly, the residents said that they would prefer a concise, point-by-point presentation of the Essential Facts of each case in an easy-to-read, bulleted format. This approach is easy on exhausted eyes and provides a quick review of Pearls and Pitfalls as information is absorbed during repeated study sessions. We worked hard to choose cases that could be presented well in this format, recognizing the limitations inherent in reproducing high-quality images in print. Unlike the authors of other case-based radiology review books, we removed the guesswork by providing clear annotations and descriptions for all images. In our opinion, there is nothing worse than being unable to locate a subtle finding on a poorly reproduced image even after one knows the final diagnosis.

The electronic cases expand on the printed book and provide a comprehensive review of the entire subspecialty. Thousands of cases are strategically designed to increase the resident's knowledge by providing exposure to additional case examples—from basic to advanced—and by exploring "Aunt Minnie's," unusual diagnoses, and variability within a single diagnosis. The search engine gives the resident a fighting chance to find the Holy Grail by creating individualized, daily study lists that are not limited by factors such as a radiology subsection. For example, tailor today's study list to cases involving tuberculosis and include cases in every subspecialty and every system of the body. Or study only thoracic cases, including those with links to cardiology, nuclear medicine, and pediatrics. Or study only musculoskeletal cases. The choice is yours.

As enthusiastic partners in this project, we started small and, with the encouragement, talent, and guidance of Tim Hiscock at Thieme, continued to raise the bar in our effort to assist residents in tackling the daunting task of assimilating massive amounts of information. We are passionate about continuing this journey, hoping to expand the cases in our electronic series, adapt cases based on direct feedback from residents, and increase the features intended for board review and self-assessment. As the American Board of Radiology converts its certifying examinations to an electronic format, our series will be the one best suited to meet the needs of the next generation of overworked and exhausted residents in radiology.

*Jonathan Lorenz, MD*
*Hector Ferral, MD*
Chicago, IL

# Preface

This book is not intended to teach neuroradiology—it is only a review of the most frequent pathologies and serves as a tool to be able to tell them apart. Of course, telling them apart is not always possible, and that is the whole trick of giving a pertinent set of differential diagnoses and trying to favor one over the other. Our advice is to always look at the first image and try to describe as much as you can, as if it was the only image you had available, then go through the rest of the images and see if the thought process was similar. It would be impossible to include all the pertinent differential diagnoses for each case with the format limitation of three differential diagnoses per case.

This way of teaching imaging analysis can both be similar to and very different from your daily clinical practice. Often, the pertinent finding or telltale sign to achieve a diagnosis lies in just a few of the images within an entire examination;

however, you have to see the entire case and find these. Here, images that have been deemed key by someone else are selected, giving you the advantage of a focused search but the limitation of a narrow representation. You may find yourself frustrated by offering a totally different differential diagnosis from the one presented to you here, but be aware that the same case can have a completely different approach based on the way it is presented, the order of the images, or the finding in which you are focusing your process of thought.

Additional references are provided to help you widen the scope of your review, especially in subjects that you may find more challenging or controversial.

We hope that with the interactive nature of this publication, you will have the chance to give us some feedback and help us improve and update this material on a frequent basis.

# Acknowledgments

I have to thank so many people for helping in the preparation of this book. To Santiago Restrepo for introducing us to this exciting project. To my coauthor Eliana for her support and endless drives to the island to complete cases. To all my mentors who had the patience to guide me to this point: Miguel Ruiz, Leonidas Borrero, Ramon Figueroa, Rafael Rojas, and Leonard Swischuk. I thank Dr. Faustino Guinto, who created the amazing teaching file of the University of Texas Medical Branch (UTMB) neuroradiology and taught me so many things, and Gregory Chaljub and Greg Katzman for their support.

To my colleagues in neuroradiology at UTMB, who contributed to the cases and supported me during the preparation of the material. Special thanks to all the neuroradiology fellows and residents who have inspired me on a daily basis and were the fuel to make this project a reality. Multiple medical students helped to arrange our neuroradiology teaching file, and without their effort this book would not be possible.

Some of the cases were obtained from the Medical College of Georgia, Charity Hospital in New Orleans, and The Children's Hospital in New Orleans—my thanks to everybody who contributed in our search for cases. This project would have not been possible without the support of my family, who has lived through the long hours of preparation of the material. To my parents Lucy and Roy for helping me become who I am.

To Tim Hiscock and Adriana di Giorgio at Thieme Medical Publishers for their everlasting patience.

Thank you.

—*Roy Riascos*

I have immense gratitude for my partner Roy Riascos for inviting me on this stimulating journey. This project would have not been possible without all of the help from my mentors and supportive colleagues, or without the forgiveness and patience of my loving family. Two of my professors departed, but the drive and wisdom that they gave me remained. God bless Dr. Edwin D. Cacayorin and Dr. Joel Yeakley. I thank Leo Hochhauser, Clark Sitton, Emilio Supsupin, and Alex Simonetta, my benevolent colleagues, who have been strengthening our department, contributing to the teaching file, and continuously encouraging me with this endeavor. I thank my Colombian teachers, Anibal Morillo, Maria Isabel Mantilla, and Sonia Bermudez, who opened up my mind to this fascinating world of neuroradiology. And of course, my beloved parents, Juan and Ester, who taught me what can be found at the other end of persistence.

—*Eliana Bonfante*

# Case 1

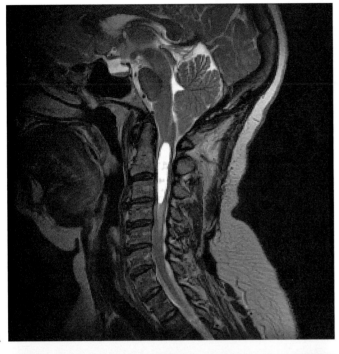

A

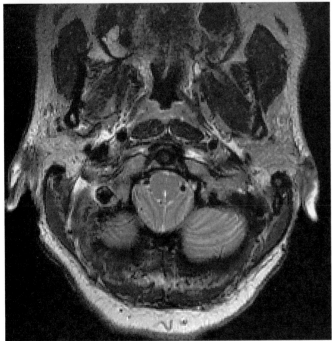

B

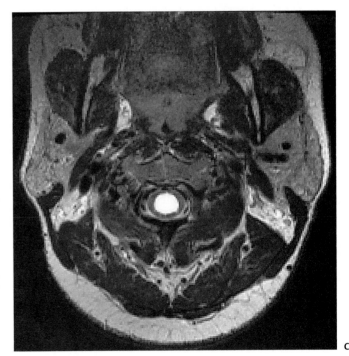

C

### ■ Clinical Presentation

A 14-year-old girl presenting with occipital headaches during Valsalva maneuver and anesthesia in both arms.

### Imaging Findings

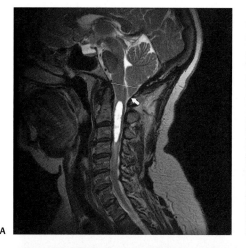

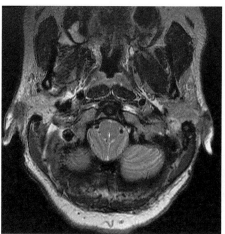

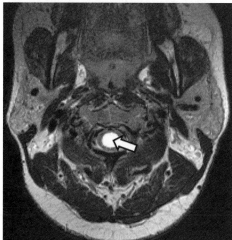

**(A)** Midsagittal T2-weighted image (WI) at the foramen magnum demonstrates a 12-mm descent of the tip of the cerebellar tonsils (*arrow*) below a line between the basion and the opisthion. A cervical syrinx is also noted. **(B)** Axial T2WI at the foramen magnum demonstrates ectopia of the cerebellar tonsils and effacement of the subarachnoid space. **(C)** Axial T2WI of the cervical spine shows a syrinx (*arrow*).

### Differential Diagnosis

- ***Chiari type I malformation:*** This patient has the typical peglike pointed tonsils displaced into the upper cervical canal with associated syringomyelia.
- *Chiari type II malformation:* Chiari type II malformation presents with deformity of the brainstem and enlargement of the foramen magnum. It is associated with myelomeningocele.
- *Spinal hypotension syndrome:* This is characterized by downward displacement of the cerebellar tonsils secondary to low pressure within the spinal canal. The brainstem and 3rd ventricle "sag" inferiorly, and the pituitary gland is upwardly convex. If contrast is administered, dural thickening and enhancement are demonstrated.

### Essential Facts

- Chiari type I malformation is defined as caudal extension of the cerebellar tonsils 5 mm below the foramen magnum.
- Syringomyelia is seen in one-half of the patients.
- It is not associated with other neurulation malformations.

- Associated anomalies are shortening of the clivus, basilar invagination, C1 assimilation, and fused cervical vertebrae (Klipper-Feil syndrome).
- Cerebrospinal fluid flow studies may be useful if the imaging findings or clinical symptoms are not typical.

### ✓ Pearls & ✗ Pitfalls

- ✓ On axial images, visualization of the cerebellar tonsils at the level of the dens is indicative of ectopia.
- ✗ Patients with long-standing compensated hydrocephalus may present with descent of the cerebellar tonsils and symptoms similar to those of patients with Chiari type I malformation.

# Case 2

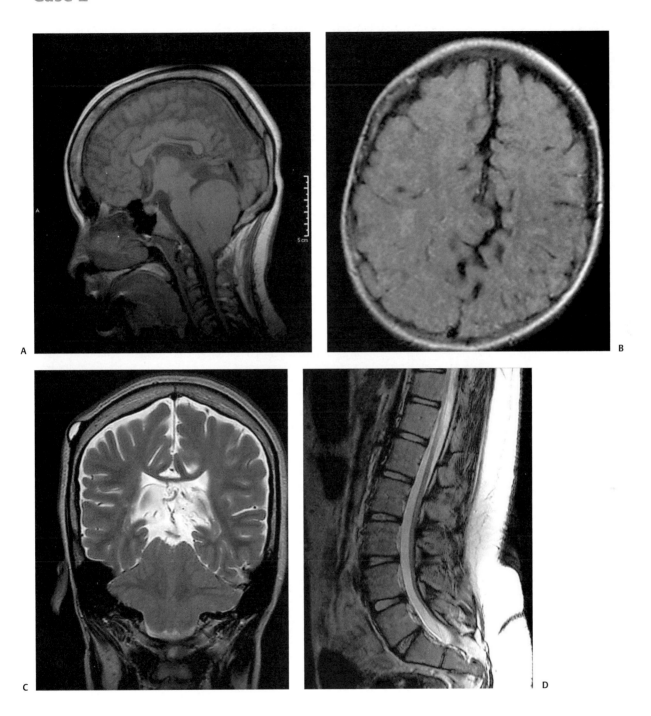

## Clinical Presentation

A 25-year-old patient initially presenting with lower extremity paralysis, respiratory distress, and impaired swallowing.

## ■ Imaging Findings

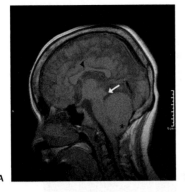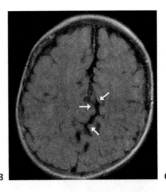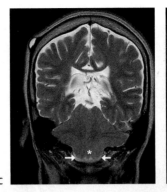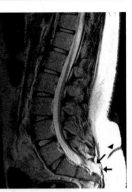

A                                   B                                   C                                   D

**(A)** Sagittal T1-weighted image (WI) of the brain shows inferior protrusion of the cerebellar vermis through a widened foramen magnum (*asterisk*). Note the tectal beaking (*arrow*) and dysgenesis of the corpus callosum (*arrowhead*). The 4th ventricle is effaced. **(B)** Axial fluid-attenuated inversion recovery image of the brain demonstrates an interdigitation of the sulci of the brain in the midline (*arrows*) secondary to hypoplasia of the cerebral falx. **(C)** Coronal T2WI of the brain shows a towering cerebellum and inferior tilting of the cerebellar tonsils through the foramen magnum (*white arrows*) along with the vermis (*asterisk*). **(D)** Sagittal T2WI of the spine shows posterior dysraphism of the sacrum (*arrows*) with an associated sinus tract (*arrowhead*).

## ■ Differential Diagnosis

These three pathologic conditions are associated with crowding of the foramen magnum:
- **Chiari type II malformation:** Chiari type II malformations are complex developmental disorders of the posterior brain that can be associated with closure defects of the neural tube, myelomeningocele, and dysgenesis of the corpus callosum.
- **Chiari type III malformation:** Chiari type III malformations have the same characteristics as Chiari type II malformations but are associated with encephalocele instead of myelomeningocele.
- **Medulloblastoma:** Medulloblastomas are malignant primitive neuroectodermal tumors of the posterior fossa that arise from the roof of the 4th ventricle. They can be similar to Chiari type II malformations, as they efface the 4th ventricle and can be isointense to the cerebellum on T1-weighted noncontrasted images. Contrast helps to differentiate them, as more than 90% of medulloblastomas enhance.

## ■ Essential Facts

- Chiari type II malformations are associated with defects of the following structures:
  - Skull: lacunar skull; concave clivus; low-riding torcula; wide foramen magnum and upper cervical canal
  - Dura: fenestrated falx causing interdigitating sulci; heart-shaped incisura; hypoplastic cerebellar tentorium
  - Posterior fossa: towering cerebellum; downward vermian displacement; slitlike 4th ventricle; tectal beaking; wrapping of cerebellum around brainstem; medullary kink
  - Other common associated defects: myelomeningocele (90%); dysgenesis of the corpus callosum (85%); hydrocephalus (75%); syringomyelia (50%); aqueductal stenosis (50%); holoprosencephaly; tethered cord

## ■ Other Imaging Findings

- Magnetic resonance imaging is the imaging modality of choice for the characterization of Chiari malformations.

## ✓ Pearls & ✗ Pitfalls

- ✓ Myelomeningocele and dysgenesis of the corpus callosum are seen in almost all cases of Chiari type II malformation.
- ✗ A complete evaluation of the spine is needed when posterior fossa defects are detected, as posterior dysraphism may not be clinically evident.
- ✗ Early detection and surgical treatment of a Chiari type II malformation will reduce the risk for permanent neurologic defect.

# Case 3

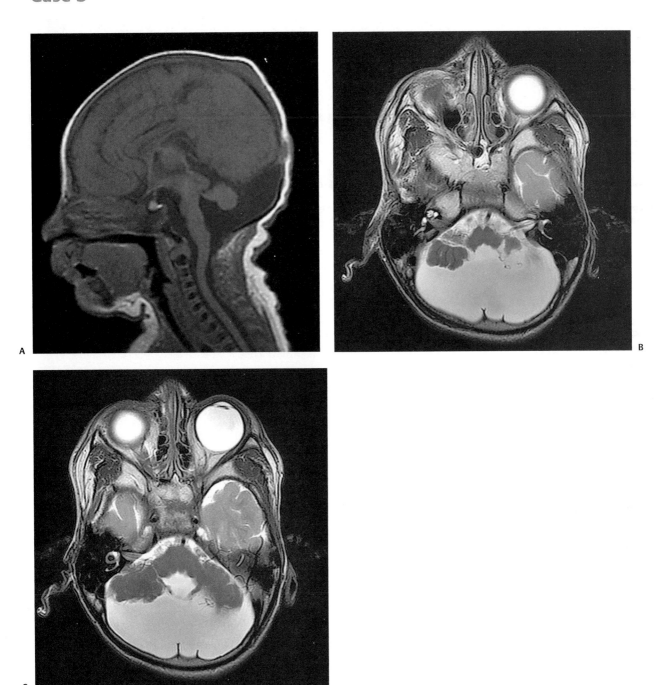

## ▪ Clinical Presentation

A 4-year-old boy with developmental delay and seizures.

### ■ Imaging Findings

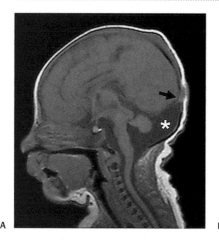 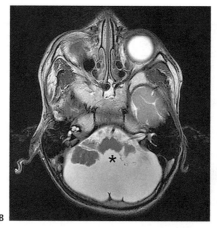 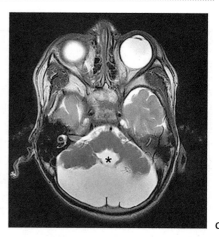

A　　　　　　　　　　B　　　　　　　　　　C

**(A)** Sagittal T1-weighted image (WI) of the brain demonstrates a large posterior fossa and an elevated insertion of the tentorium (*arrow*) with respect to the expected position. A cyst (*asterisk*) that communicates with the 4th ventricle fills the posterior fossa. **(B,C)** Axial T2WIs of the brain show cystic dilatation of the 4th ventricle (*asterisks*), which is ballooning between hypoplastic cerebellar hemispheres. The cerebellar vermis is absent.

### ■ Differential Diagnosis

- ***Dandy-Walker continuum:*** The high insertion of the tentorium and cystic dilatation of the 4th ventricle are typical features of Dandy-Walker continuum. The degree of cerebellar hypogenesis may vary.
- *Mega cisterna magna:* Enlargement of the cisterna magna and posterior fossa without abnormality in the 4th ventricle or vermis is typical of this diagnosis.
- *Arachnoid cyst:* The 4th ventricle and vermis are normal but displaced by the cyst.

### ■ Essential Facts

- An enlarged posterior fossa and a high position of the tentorium with upward displacement of the lateral sinuses and torcular Herophili are common in Dandy-Walker continuum.
- Varying degrees of cerebellar agenesis or hypogenesis are seen.
- As a result of cystic dilatation of the 4th ventricle, it fills nearly the entire posterior fossa.
- Cerebellar hypoplasia: hypogenesis of the cerebellar vermis and cystic dilatation of the 4th ventricle without posterior fossa enlargement were formerly known as Dandy-Walker variant.
- Associated anomalies, present in 70% of cases, include the following:
  - Agenesis of the corpus callosum, migration anomalies, cephalocele, holoprosencephaly, hydrocephalus, and porencephaly, among others

### ✓ Pearls & ✗ Pitfalls

- ✓ Conditions associated with abnormal cerebellar size:
  - Cerebellar atrophy: the cerebellum is small and the cerebellar fissures are enlarged.
  - Cerebellar hypoplasia: the cerebellum is small, but the fissures are normal in size compared with the folia.
  - Cerebellar dysplasia: disorganized development; an abnormal folial pattern ranging from absence of fissures to large folia with shallow fissures to foliation in abnormal directions or heterotopic nodules of gray matter may be present.
  - Cerebellar hypogenesis: the superior portions of the cerebellum are formed, but the inferior portions are not; this term should not be used because it overlaps with dysplasia.
- ✗ An isolated 4th ventricle, which is the result of obstruction of both the aqueduct of Sylvius and the 4th ventricular outflow foramina, may give the appearance of a hypoplastic cerebellum. The lateral and 3rd ventricles appear slightly enlarged or normal if there is a functioning ventriculoperitoneal shunt. The distal aqueduct may be enlarged.

# Case 4

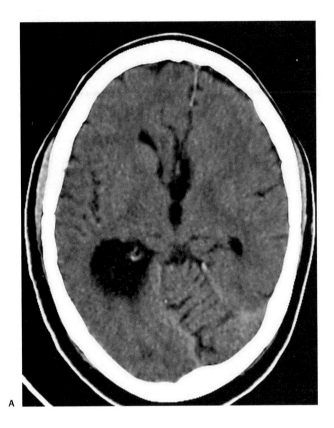

A

## ▣ Clinical Presentation

A 12-year-old boy with slight cognitive defects.

## Further Work-up

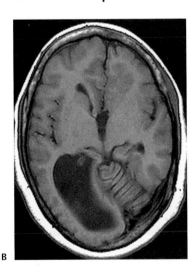

B

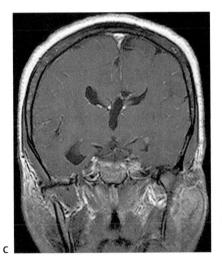

C

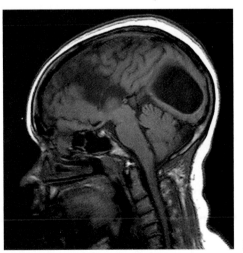

D

### ■ Imaging Findings

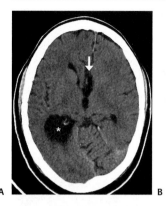 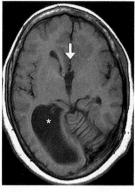 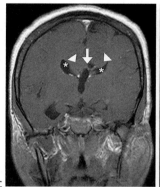 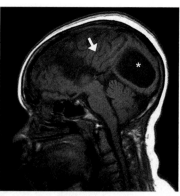

A    B    C    D

**(A)** Axial computed tomography (CT) scan of the head shows an absence of the anterior fibers of the corpus callosum (*arrow*) and a dilated lateral ventricle on the right (*asterisk*). **(B)** Axial T1-weighted magnetic resonance (MR) image of the brain shows an absence of the anterior fibers of the corpus callosum (*arrow*) and a dilated lateral ventricle on the right (*asterisk*). **(C)** Coronal T1-weighted image (WI) of the brain after intravenous contrast shows absence of the corpus callosum with a high-riding 3rd ventricle (*arrow*). Note the "bullhorns" appearance of the lateral horns (*asterisks*). Thick bands of white matter superior to the lateral ventricles are Probst fibers (*arrowheads*). **(D)** Sagittal T1WI of the brain shows absence of the corpus callosum. Note the lack of a cingulate gyrus, the vertically oriented sulci (*arrow*), and the colpocephaly of the right lateral ventricle (*asterisk*).

### ■ Differential Diagnosis

- **Dysgenesis of the corpus callosum (CC):** This is suggested by partial or complete absence of the CC.
- *Lobar holoprosencephaly:* Partial agenesis of the CC can be seen in lobar holoprosencephaly. Other findings include fusion of anterior horns and lateral ventricles and fusion of the anterior fornix. There is an absence of septum pellucidum. This entity is associated with midline facial defects. There is no thalamic fusion (seen in more severe forms of holoprosencephaly).
- *Schizencephaly:* This is a migration disorder that can be associated with partial dysplasia of the CC. The main findings include hemispheric cerebrospinal fluid–filled clefts through which the ventricles communicate with the subpial space. The clefts are lined by gray matter. Unilateral schizencephaly is more frequent than bilateral defects.

### ■ Essential Facts

- Bundles of Probst: tracks of white matter that run parallel to the ventricle as an alternative to the CC
- High-riding 3rd ventricle
- Absent cingulate sulcus with radially oriented fissures
- Crescent-shaped lateral horns; small ("bullhorns") appearance of the frontal horns
- Enlarged occipital horns (colpocephaly)
- Absence of the septum pellucidum or severe widening of the cavum septum pellucidum
- The precursors of the CC develop between 8 and 20 weeks. Many different genes control the movement of axons across the midline, and numerous mutations can result in callosal defects.
- The CC develops from the anterior genu to the posterior splenium. The rostrum is the last portion to develop.

- Associated with other central nervous system anomalies: anomalies of cortical development, lipoma or interhemispheric cyst, Dandy-Walker complex, Chiari type II malformation, encephalocele (midfacial anomalies), and holoprosencephaly
- Sagittal and coronal MR imaging of the brain is the best diagnostic tool for this condition.

### ■ Other Imaging Findings

- Fetal ultrasound after week 20 can detect severe callosal defects.
- Partial callosal agenesis can be hard to detect on ultrasound.

### ✓ Pearls & ✗ Pitfalls

- ✓ Lipomas of the midline associated with agenesis of the CC calcify in 10% of cases and are seen on CT.
- ✓ Callosal agenesis is the most common finding in fetal alcohol syndrome.
- ✗ In patients with an enlarged 3rd ventricle secondary to hydrocephalus, evaluation of the CC is limited because of the thinning and superior displacement of the fibers. Wait until the ventricles are decompressed before undertaking further assessment.
- ✗ When all the segments of the CC are present but small, the condition is considered to be callosal hypoplasia.

# Case 5

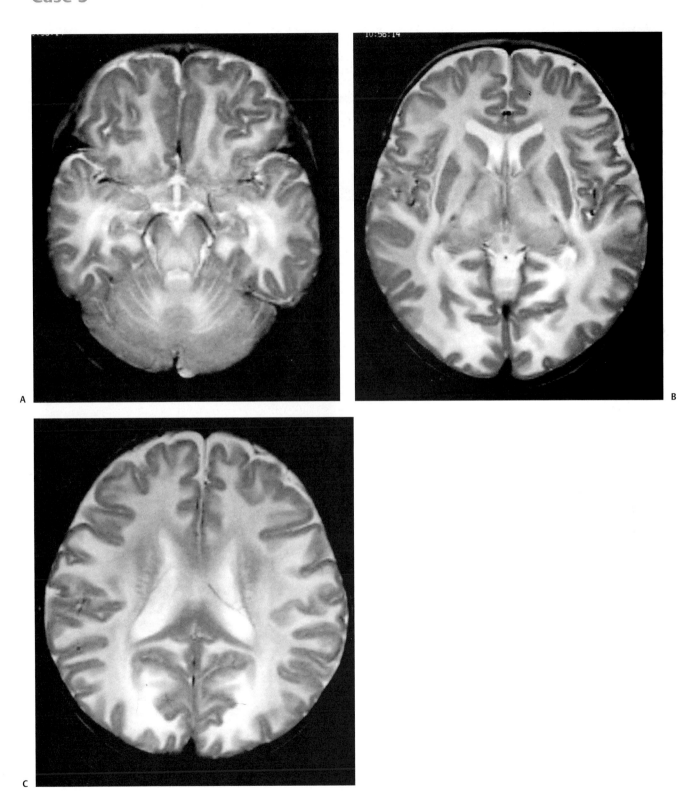

A

B

C

■ **Clinical Presentation**

An infant presenting with marked hypotonia, macrocephaly, and seizures.

### ■ Imaging Findings

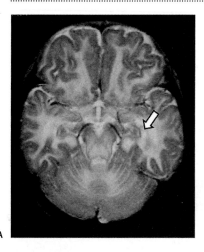 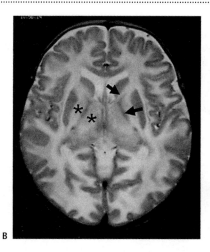 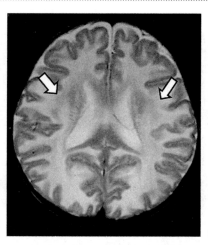

**(A)** Axial T2-weighted magnetic resonance (MR) image of the brain reveals an increased white matter T2 signal (*arrow*). **(B)** There is relative sparing of the internal capsule (*arrows*). Abnormal T2 signal is demonstrated in the thalami (*asterisks*) and globus pallidus. **(C)** Note the diffuse increase in the white matter T2 signal (*arrows*).

### ■ Differential Diagnosis

• **Canavan disease:** This involves predominantly the subcortical U fibers. The occipital lobes are more involved than the frontal and parietal lobes. The thalami and basal ganglia are affected in severe cases.
• *Alexander disease:* This also presents with macrocephaly but mostly involves frontal white matter. The affected areas may show enhancement.
• *Pelizaeus-Merzbacher disease, connatal type:* This presents with a nearly total lack of myelination. The brainstem, diencephalon, cerebellum, and subcortical white matter may demonstrate myelin preservation.

### ■ Essential Facts

• Autosomal-recessive condition, most common in Ashkenazi Jews
• Deficiency of aspartoacylase
• Hypotonia, macrocephaly, and seizures in newborn period
• Spasticity, optic atrophy, and intellectual failure as disease progresses
• Death usually by second year of life
• Computed tomography: diffuse low attenuation in cerebral and cerebellar white matter
• MR imaging: White matter has high T2 and low T1 signal. The thalami and basal ganglia can be affected.
• The peripheral white matter is preferentially affected early in the course of the disease.
• In severe cases, there may be an extensive lack of myelination with relative sparing of the internal capsules.

### ■ Other Imaging Findings

• MR spectroscopy may reveal an increased *N*-acetylaspartate (NAA) peak. Because of the deficiency in aspartoacylase, NAA accumulates in the mitochondria and impairs myelin synthesis.
• Myoinositol elevation due to gliosis may also be present.

### ✓ Pearls & ✗ Pitfalls

✓ As opposed to Canavan disease, Krabbe disease and metachromatic leukodystrophy involve the deep white matter early, and the peripheral white matter is affected as the disease progresses.

✗ In infants born prematurely, myelination may be delayed for the corrected gestational age, mimicking leukodystrophy. Adequate clinical correlation and follow-up imaging are helpful to make the distinction.

# Case 6

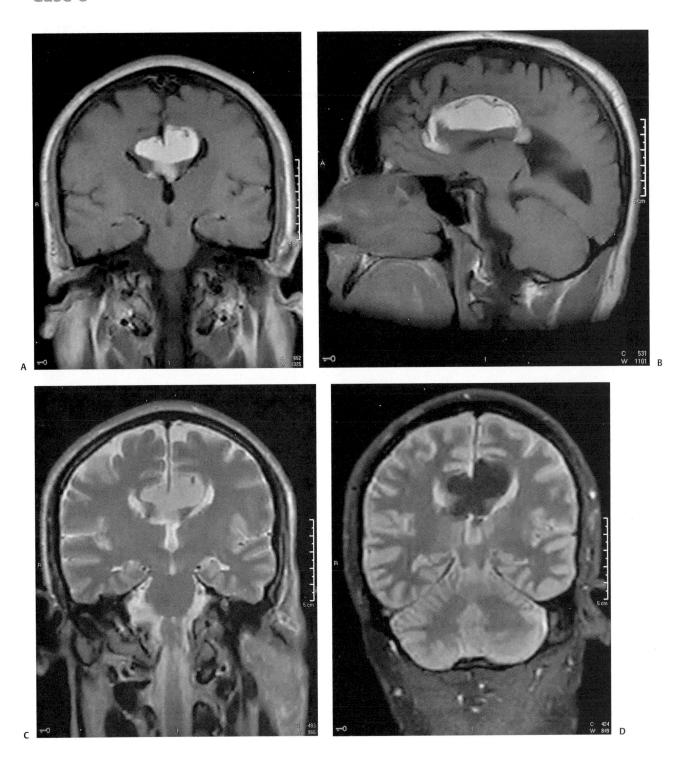

## ■ Clinical Presentation

A 30-year-old man with a history of headaches.

### ■ Imaging Findings

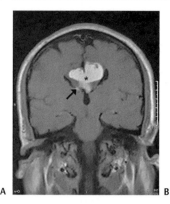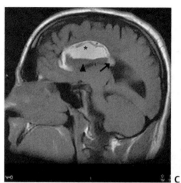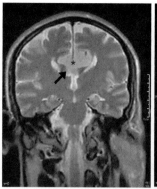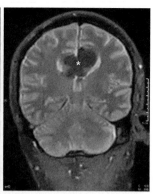

**(A)** Coronal T1-weighted magnetic resonance imaging (MRI) of the brain demonstrates a high-signal lesion in the midline (*asterisk*) at the site of the corpus callosum. The lesion shows ventricular extension (*arrow*). **(B)** Sagittal T1-weighted MRI of the brain demonstrates a high-signal lesion in the midline (*asterisk*) that shows ventricular extension (*arrow*). Note the hypoplasia of the corpus callosum (*arrowhead*). **(C)** Coronal T2-weighted MRI of the brain demonstrates a high-signal lesion in the midline (*asterisk*) at the site of the corpus callosum. The lesion shows ventricular extension (*arrow*). **(D)** Coronal T2-weighted fat-saturated MRI of the brain demonstrates loss of signal in the midline lesion (*asterisk*), which was bright before fat saturation.

### ■ Differential Diagnosis

- **Intracranial lipoma:** Intracranial lipomas are fatty, extra-axial, pia-based lesions. Calcifications are common in lesions with an interhemispheric location. They may encase vessels. Pericallosal lipomas are associated with choroidal extension. Fat suppression can aid the diagnosis.
- *Dermoid cyst:* Dermoid cysts are usually located near the parasellar or frontal region at the midline. They are well circumscribed and contain fat. Twenty percent have capsular calcification (lipomas at this location rarely calcify). Rupture of a dermoid cyst causes chemical meningitis and leptomeningeal enhancement (lipomas typically do not rupture).
- *Epidermoid cyst (ectodermal inclusion cyst):* Epidermoid cysts are lobulated. They are unusual at the midline. Fifty percent occur at the cerebellopontine angle (CPA), 17% are located at the 4th ventricle, and 10% are parasellar. On T1- and T2-weighted images, they are isointense to cerebrospinal fluid. They have a dirty fluid-attenuated inversion recovery signal. These cysts restrict on diffusion (this feature is diagnostic).

### ■ Essential Facts

- Poor differentiation of the embryonic meninx primitiva (forms leptomeninges and cisterns), then differentiation into fat
- Locations in order of frequency: interhemispheric (40–45%), suprasellar-infundibular (25%), quadrigeminal cistern (25%), and CPA (14%)
- Associated with other malformations
- When associated with dysgenesis of the corpus callosum (interhemispheric), described as tubulonodular type
- Cephaloceles

### ■ Other Imaging Findings

- Computed tomography can identify calcifications.
- Lipomas are suppressed on fat-saturated MRI.
- Magnetic resonance spectroscopy will show a high lipid peak.

### ✓ Pearls & ✗ Pitfalls

- ✓ There are two types of pericallosal lipomas: bulky (tubulonodular), which are associated with agenesis of the corpus callosum, and ribbon-like (curvilinear).
- ✗ Other entities with a high T1 signal:
  - Hemorrhage
    - Early subacute (3–7 days): intracellular methemoglobin
    - Late subacute (7–14 days): extracellular methemoglobin
  - Lesions with a high protein content
  - Melanin
  - Lipids
  - Minerals (manganesium)
  - Slow flow

# Case 7

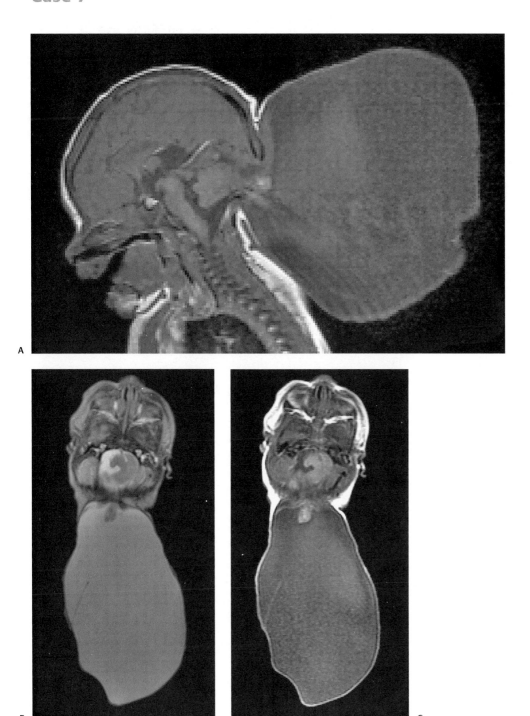

## ▣ Clinical Presentation

A newborn with a posterior neck mass diagnosed on prenatal ultrasound.

### Imaging Findings

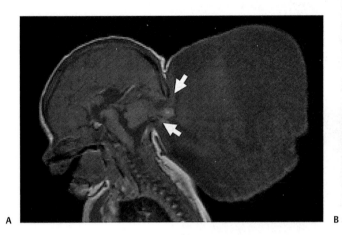 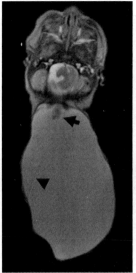 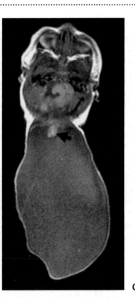

**(A)** Sagittal T1-weighted image of the brain shows a posterior skull defect (*arrows*) through which cerebellar tissue and cerebrospinal fluid are protruding. **(B)** Axial T2WI of the brain demonstrates elongation of the cerebellum, which protrudes toward the neck (*arrow*) and is surrounded by a large cystic lesion. Note a thin septum within the cyst (*arrowhead*). **(C)** Axial T1WI of the brain demonstrates elongation of the cerebellum, which protrudes toward the neck (*arrow*) and is surrounded by a large cystic lesion.

### Differential Diagnosis

- ***Occipital meningoencephalocele:*** In occipital meningoencephalocele, there is posterior traction of the cerebellum. The cystic lesion communicates with the subarachnoid space of the posterior fossa.
- *Chiari type III malformation:* Chiari type III malformation has the same features as a Chiari type II malformation, but with an occipital cephalocele instead of a myelomeningocele. This patient's brainstem is not elongated.
- *Cystic hygroma:* Although hygromas may be unilocular, they involve the neck, oral cavity, face, or airway as well as surrounding normal muscles. No skull defect is present.

### Essential Facts

- Occipital cephaloceles originate between the foramen magnum and the lambda and have variable contents. The brain within them is usually dysplastic, gliotic cerebellum.
- Associated anomalies include Chiari type II and III malformations, Dandy-Walker complex, cerebellar dysplasias, diastematomyelia, and Klippel-Feil syndrome.

### Other Imaging Findings

- Ultrasound may detect occipital meningoencephaloceles early in pregnancy.
- Computed tomography demonstrates the bony defects.

### ✓ Pearls & ✗ Pitfalls

- ✓ For the purposes of surgical planning, it is important to identify the position of the venous sinuses and the presence of associated brain anomalies.
- ✗ Occipital cephaloceles without brainstem anomalies are often mislabeled as Chiari type III malformations.

# Case 8

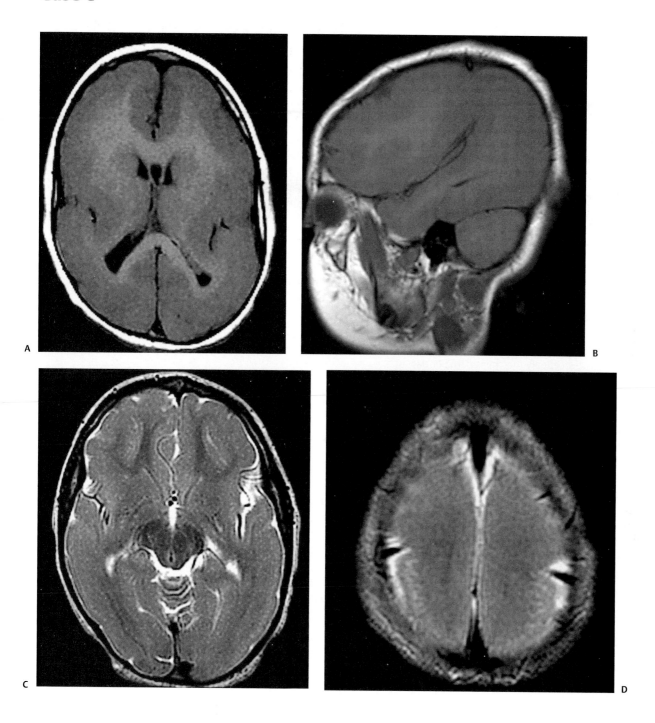

A

B

C

D

## ▦ Clinical Presentation

.....................................................................................................................................................................

A 2-year-old girl presenting with developmental delay and seizures.

### ■ Imaging Findings

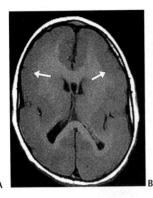 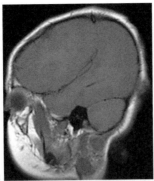 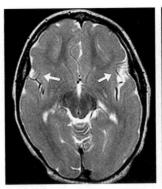 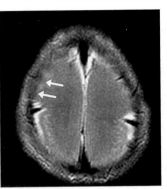

**(A)** Axial T1-weighted image (WI) shows severely decreased sulcation of the brain with a thick cortex (*arrows*). **(B)** Sagittal T1WI shows a thick cortical layer with severely decreased sulcation. **(C)** Axial T2WI shows severely decreased sulcation of the brain with a thick cortex (*arrows*). **(D)** Axial T2WI shows severely decreased sulcation of the brain with a thick cortex (*arrows*).

### ■ Differential Diagnosis

- **Type I (classic) lissencephaly:** Type I lissencephaly is a migration disorder of the gray matter, with the formation of a smooth, four-layered cortex (a normal cortex has six layers). Type I lissencephaly may be isolated or part of a syndrome, most frequently Miller-Dieker syndrome.
- **Type II lissencephaly (cobblestone complex):** Type II lissencephaly has a disorganized, unlayered cortex and no ribbons of band heterotopia. Neurons migrate past the cortical plate to the subpial space. No subependymal heterotopia should be present. Type II lissencephaly is associated with congenital muscular dystrophy (Walker-Warburg syndrome). Ocular defects are common.
- **Cytomegalovirus (CMV) infection:** Cortical gyral abnormalities, including lissencephaly, can be seen in CMV infections. Other findings include microcephaly, cerebral periventricular and parenchymal calcifications, and cerebellar hypoplasia.

### ■ Essential Facts

- Type I lissencephaly is part of the agyria/pachygyria spectrum (hourglass configuration of brain).
- In the usual presentation, the outer cortex exhibits ribbons of band heterotopia separated by white matter.
- Subependymal heterotopia is commonly seen.
- There is no abnormal enhancement.
- Fetal ultrasound can detect severe cases of subependymal heterotopia.

### ■ Other Imaging Findings

- Diffusion tensor tracking has shown a band of anisotropic diffusion related to the dysplastic 4th cortical layer and a disconnection between the cortex and the deep white matter.

### ✓ Pearls & ✗ Pitfalls

- ✓ Always look for other sites of heterotopic cortex. Some enhancement has been described at the dense cellular layer (dysplastic cortical layer). Remember that a smooth cortex can be seen in normal fetuses until up to 26 weeks of gestation.
- ✗ Multiple migration disorders can appear similar to lissencephaly.
- ✗ Knowledge of the gestational age is important to avoid overcalling agyria.
- ✗ Only magnetic resonance imaging late in pregnancy can detect lissencephaly in utero.

# Case 9

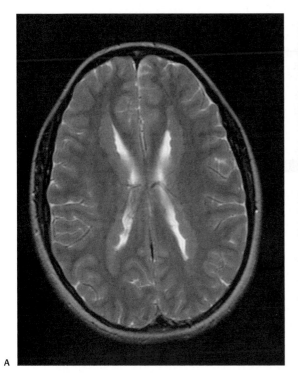 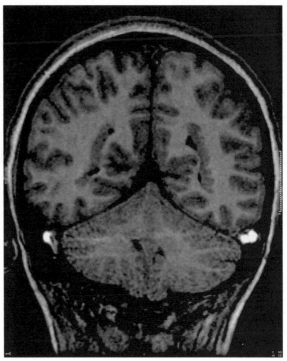

A                                                                                          B

## ◼ Clinical Presentation

A patient undergoing a work-up for epilepsy.

### ■ Imaging Findings

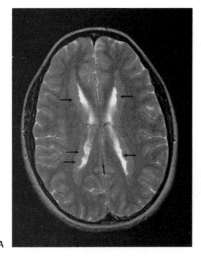
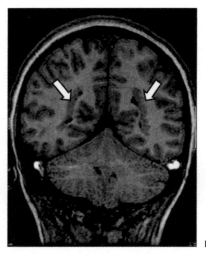

**(A)** Axial T2-weighted image (WI) of the brain demonstrates multiple nodules, with signal intensity similar to that of the cerebral cortex, lining the lateral ventricles (*arrows*). There is a serrated appearance of the inner margin of the ventricles. **(B)** Coronal T1WI confirms the presence of nodules along the ventricular walls. The nodules have signal intensity like that of the cortex (*arrows*).

### ■ Differential Diagnosis

- ***Subependymal heterotopia:*** Nodules of gray matter along the ventricular surface are suggestive of subependymal heterotopia. This may appear exophytic, extending to the ventricle.
- *Subependymal nodules of tuberous sclerosis:* These are irregularly shaped and often calcified. They are not isointense to cortex. They may enhance.
- *Band heterotopia:* Band heterotopia appears as homogeneous bands of gray matter between the lateral ventricles and cerebral cortex, separated from both by layers of normal-appearing white matter.

### ■ Essential Facts

- Heterotopia: arrest of the radial migration of neurons, leading to ectopic neurons in areas other than the cortex
- Three types
  - Subependymal
    - Normal development; seizures
    - Smooth, ovoid masses isointense to gray matter in all sequences
  - Focal subcortical
    - Motor and intellectual disturbance, epilepsy
    - Large heterogeneous mass, isointense to cortical gray matter
    - The affected hemisphere is small with thin cortex and shallow sulci.
    - Associated hypogenesis of the corpus callosum and dysplastic basal ganglia
  - Band (laminar) heterotopia
    - Considered a mild form of classic lissencephaly
    - Variable developmental delay and seizures
    - Female preponderance (90%)
    - Homogeneous bands of gray matter between the lateral ventricles and cerebral cortex, separated from both by a layer of normal-appearing white matter
    - May have foci of high T2 signal in the white matter

### ■ Other Imaging Findings

- On positron emission tomography with fluorodeoxyglucose, band heterotopia has glucose uptake similar to or greater than that of normal cortex. This contrasts with the hypometabolism found in cortical dysplasias.

### ✓ Pearls & ✗ Pitfalls

- ✓ Lesions may not be apparent in infants and do not become noticeable until myelination has reached an advanced stage.
- ✗ The caudate tail along the lateral wall of the lateral ventricles should not be misinterpreted as ectopic gray matter.

# Case 10

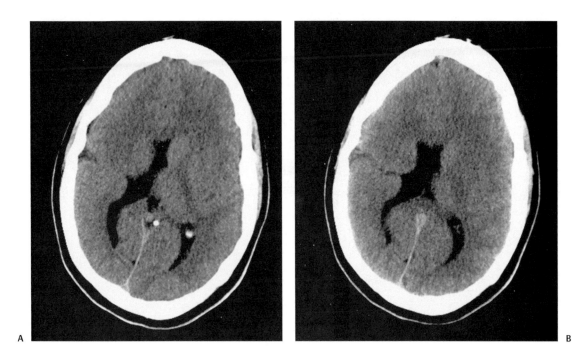

A

B

## ■ Clinical Presentation

A patient with a history of developmental delay and seizures.

## Further Work-up

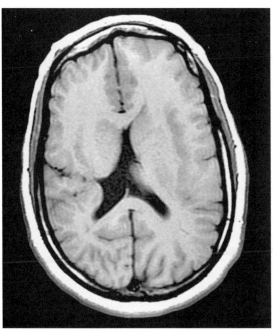

C

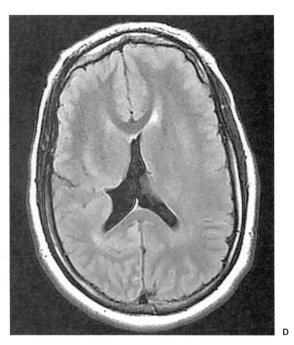

D

### ■ Imaging Findings

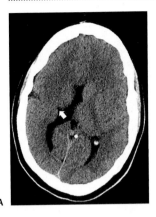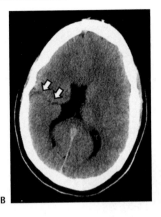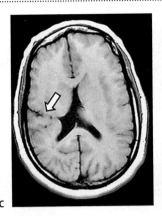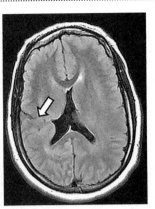

A  B  C  D

**(A)** Axial computed tomography scan of the brain demonstrates a small outpouching of the lateral wall of the right lateral ventricle, lined by gray matter (*arrow*). A deep sulcus is noted in the subjacent cortex. **(B)** A contiguous slice demonstrates a cleft with cerebrospinal fluid (CSF) attenuation through which the lateral ventricle communicates with the subarachnoid space. The defect is lined by gray matter (*arrows*). **(C)** Axial T1-weighted image of the brain show a CSF-filled cleft, lined by gray matter, between the subarachnoid space and the lateral wall of the right lateral ventricle (*arrow*). **(D)** Axial fluid-attenuated inversion recovery image of the brain shows a CSF-filled cleft, lined by gray matter, between the subarachnoid space and the lateral wall of the right lateral ventricle (*arrow*).

### ■ Differential Diagnosis

- **Closed-lip schizencephaly:** Closed-lip schizencephaly presents with a CSF cleft, lined by gray matter, that extends from the ependymal surface of the brain to the pia, with apposition of the cleft walls.
- *Focal transmantle dysplasia:* Focal transmantle dysplasia presents with abnormal cells extending from the cortex to the ventricular surface, seen as a curvilinear focus of hyperintensity relative to the mature white matter. No CSF-filled cleft is present.
- *Band heterotopia:* The abnormally positioned bands of gray matter are parallel in band heterotopia, not perpendicular to the ventricular walls, and are not surrounded by CSF.

### ■ Essential Facts

- Schizencephaly is an anomaly of neuronal migration in which a CSF-filled cleft is lined by gray matter. It extends from the ventricular surface (ependyma) to the periphery (pial surface) of the brain.
- Types
  - Closed-lip (type I) schizencephaly: cleft walls in apposition, with a ventricular dimple
  - Open-lip (type II) schizencephaly: cleft walls separated (more common)
- Polymicrogyric and nonpolymicrogyric cleft linings, cystlike diverticula and membranous structures, and subependymal heterotopia can be found at the cleft
- Concomitant anomalies are polymicrogyria outside the cleft, white matter volume loss, septal and optic anomalies, callosal anomalies, and hippocampal anomalies.

### ✓ Pearls & ✗ Pitfalls

- ✓ A thin pial membrane covers the cerebral defect in schizencephaly. It separates the cleft from the subarachnoid space.
- ✗ A cleft with closed lips in the imaging plane may be missed. At least two planes are necessary to assess patients with seizure or developmental delay.

# Case 11

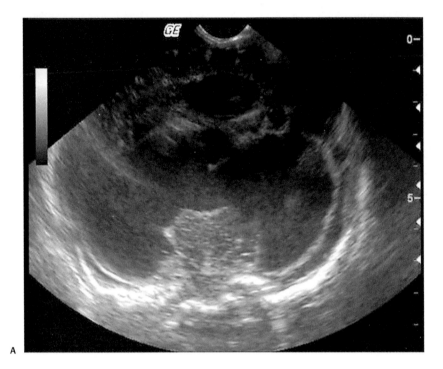

A

## Clinical Presentation

A newborn infant with feeding problems and seizures. The baby has a cleft lip.

## Further Work-up

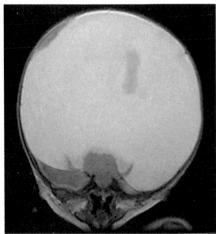

B

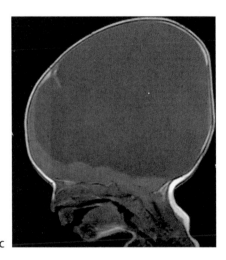

C

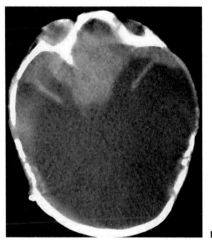

D

## ■ Imaging Findings

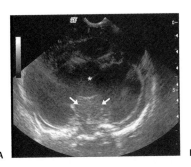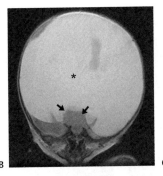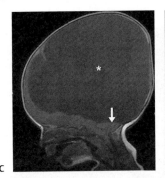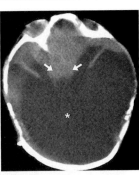

A                                   B                                   C                                   D

**(A)** Transfontanellar ultrasound of the brain in a coronal view at the level of the thalami shows a prominent monoventricle (*asterisk*) and thalamic fusion (*arrows*). **(B)** Coronal T2-weighted magnetic resonance image of the brain at the level of the thalami shows a monoventricle, seen as a prominent supratentorial cyst (*asterisk*), and fusion of the thalami (*arrows*). Note the absence of a cerebral falx. **(C)** Sagittal T1-weighted image of the brain shows a large supratentorial cyst (*asterisk*); note the hypoplasia of the posterior fossa structures (*arrow*). **(D)** Axial computed tomography scan of the brain without contrast shows fusion of the thalami (*arrows*) and a large posterior cyst-monoventricle (*asterisk*).

## ■ Differential Diagnosis

- **Alobar holoprosencephaly:** Alobar holoprosencephaly is a congenital malformation of the forebrain. The corpus callosum is absent. There is a dorsal cyst with hydrocephalus. Macrocephaly can arise from high pressure. The anterior brain is compressed anteriorly, and the thalami are fused.
- *Hydranencephaly:* Intrauterine destruction of the cerebral hemispheres secondary to occlusion of the internal carotid arteries is called hydranencephaly. The thalami are not fused as in holoprosencephaly. The cerebral falx is intact. Macrocrania is also noted. The posterior fossa structures are intact, and there is absence of a cortical mantle.
- *Severe (obstructive) hydrocephalus:* There is increased cerebrospinal fluid formation versus insufficient resorption in severe hydrocephalus. Macrocrania can develop if severe hydrocephalus occurs early in life, when the sutures are open. The compressed brain has a cortical mantle appearance (characteristic) not seen in holoprosencephaly. No thalamic fusion is present. The site of the obstruction should be located. There is a high T2 signal in the periventricular white matter, which is not seen in holoprosencephaly or hydranencephaly.

## ■ Essential Facts

- Alobar holoprosencephaly is the most severe form of a defect in dorsoventral patterning and cleavage of the forebrain.
- The hypothalamus and caudate nuclei are the most severely affected structures.
- Azygos anterior cerebral artery can be present.

- Complex facial malformations are associated with this condition:
  - Cleft lip/palate
  - Hypotelorism
  - Arhinencephaly
  - Cyclopia
- Three types of appearance have been described for the remaining brain: "cup," "pancake," and "ball."

## ✓ Pearls & ✗ Pitfalls

- ✓ "The face predicts the brain": if facial malformations are present, the brain must be studied.
- ✓ Absence of the falx and thalamic fusion are the most relevant imaging findings.
- ✓ Facial changes are not associated with hydranencephaly or severe hydrocephalus.
- ✗ Macrocephaly can be seen in the three entities in the differential diagnosis.

# Case 12

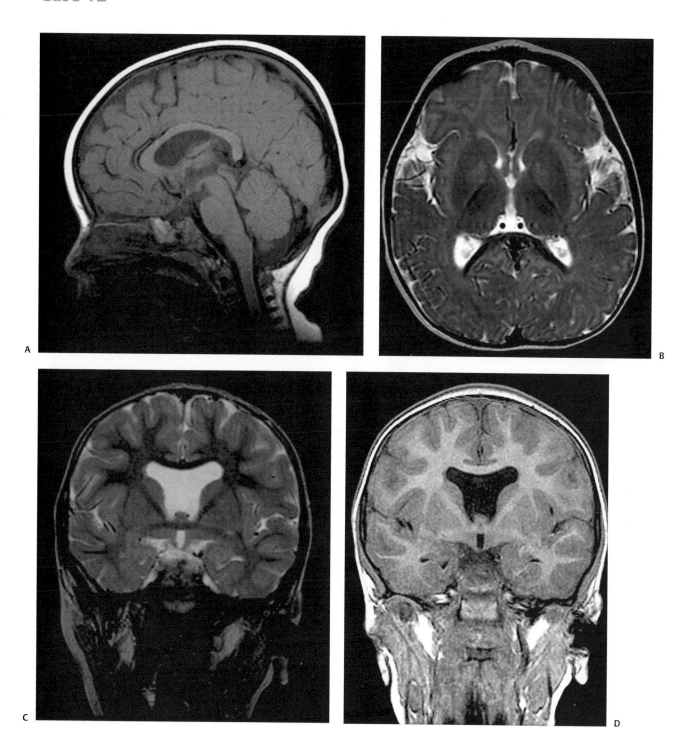

A

B

C

D

## ▪ Clinical Presentation

A 20-year-old man with a history of bilaterally decreased eyesight and hypopituitarism.

## Imaging Findings

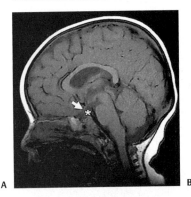
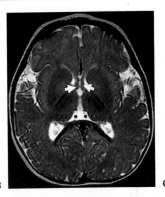
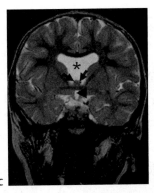
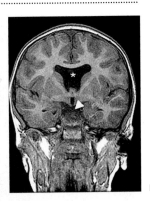

A        B        C        D

**(A)** A T1-weighted sagittal image of the brain shows a small optic chiasm (*arrow*) and absence of the pituitary stalk (*asterisk*). **(B)** A T2-weighted axial image of the brain shows two separate anterior horns of the fornix (*arrows*). **(C)** A T2-weighted sagittal image of the brain shows absence of the septum pellucidum (*asterisk*). Note the lack of fusion of the fornix (*arrows*) and the hypoplastic sella, with no evidence of a pituitary gland or pituitary stalk. Hypoplasia of the optic nerves is seen (*arrowhead*). **(D)** A T2-weighted sagittal image of the brain shows absence of the septum pellucidum (*asterisk*). Note the hypoplastic sella, with no evidence of a pituitary gland or pituitary stalk. Hypoplasia of the optic chiasm is seen (*arrowhead*).

## Differential Diagnosis

- **Septo-optic dysplasia (de Morsier syndrome):** Septo-optic dysplasia is considered the mildest form of holoprosencephaly. It is caused by dysgenesis of the septum pellucidum. The following may be present: optic nerve hypoplasia, hypothalamic and pituitary dysfunction (60% of cases), schizencephaly (50% of cases), thin corpus callosum, and square frontal horns.
- *Lobar holoprosencephaly:* A fused anterior fornix is the main feature in the brain that differentiates lobar holoprosencephaly from septo-optic dysplasia. There is an absence of the corpus callosum. This diagnosis is associated with midline defects, which are rarely seen in septo-optic dysplasia. The optic nerves and hypothalamus are spared.
- *Partial agenesis of the corpus callosum:* Here, absence of the septum pellucidum or severe widening of the cavum septum pellucidum can be seen. The optic nerves and hypothalamus are intact.

## Essential Facts

- Two distinct forms of septo-optic dysplasia are described:
  - Associated with schizencephaly: usually, a remnant of the septum pellucidum is present.
  - White matter hypoplasia, including optic radiations. There is no schizencephaly. Hypopituitarism may be present.
- Magnetic resonance imaging:
  - Best diagnostic tool
  - Thin slices through the optic nerves are helpful.

## Other Imaging Findings

- Computed tomography can detect absence of the septum pellucidum but has less contrast for visualizing migrational disorders. Evaluation of the optic tract is limited.
- It is difficult to identify findings on prenatal ultrasound.

## ✓ Pearls & ✗ Pitfalls

- ✓ The anterior fusion of the fornix helps to differentiate lobar holoprosencephaly from septo-optic dysplasia.
- ✓ Always look for schizencephaly.
- ✗ If dysgenesis or absence of the septum pellucidum is detected, investigate further to exclude septo-optic dysplasia or lobar holoprosencephaly.

# Case 13

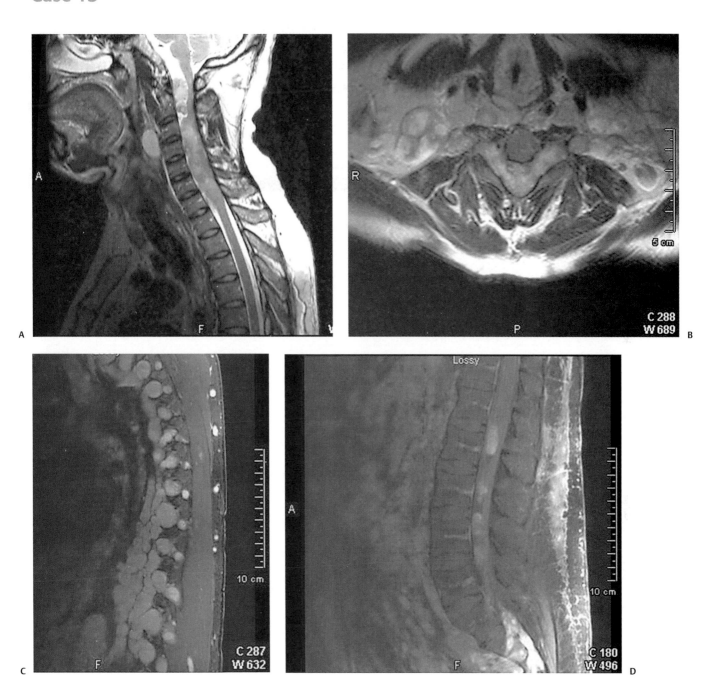

## ■ Clinical Presentation

A 40-year-old man with progressive weakness of both upper extremities for 1 year.

### ■ Imaging Findings

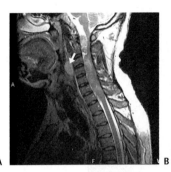
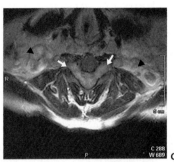
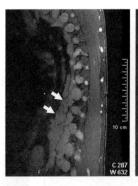
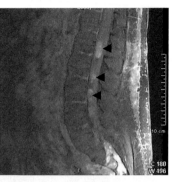

**(A)** Sagittal T2-weighted image (WI) of the cervical spine demonstrates a widened spinal canal with an intradural, extraspinal mass that compresses the spinal cord posteriorly (*arrowhead*). A soft-tissue mass in the prevertebral soft tissues shows a high T2 signal (*arrow*). **(B)** Axial T2WI of the spine at the level of C5 shows anterior compression of the spinal cord (*black arrow*) by a hyperintense, lobulated mass that occupies the spinal canal and extends through the neural foramina to the paraspinal soft tissues (*arrowheads*). Note the widening of the neural foramina (*white arrows*). **(C)** Parasagittal fat-saturated T1WI of the thoracic spine with gadolinium shows enhancing masses (*arrowheads*) at multiple levels that widen the neural foramina and extend to the paraspinal soft tissues (*arrows*). **(D)** Sagittal fat-saturated T1WI shows multiple oval, enhancing masses in the spinal canal (*arrowheads*).

### ■ Differential Diagnosis

- ***Spinal neurofibromatosis type 1 (NF1; also known as von Recklinghausen disease):*** Scoliosis is seen in 71% of cases. Plexiform neurofibromas are pathognomonic for NF1; they can have a dumbbell appearance if located in a neural foramen, which they can enlarge. They typically enhance.
- *Spinal meningioma:* Spinal meningioma appears as an enhancing mass in the spinal canal. If an extradural mass is located in the lateral and posterior aspects of the spinal canal, it is likely a meningioma, not a neurofibroma. Meningiomas do not usually extend through the neural foramen. A "dural tail" is seen in one-third of cases and is not present in neurofibromas.
- *Traumatic lateral meningocele:* Meningocele is secondary to traction on nerve root sleeves. There is usually associated traumatic injury. Look for avulsion of the nerve roots. A meningocele is a fluid-filled cavity that does not enhance. It is not associated with a soft-tissue mass or dural ectasia.

### ■ Essential Facts

- NF1 is a chromosome 17 abnormality.
- Spinal NF1 is associated with dural ectasia, lateral meningoceles, and posterior scalloping of the vertebral bodies.
- NF1 is also associated with the following:
- Plexiform neurofibromas
- Optic gliomas (30%)
- Osseous dysplasias
- Skin findings (café au lait spots, freckling, skin neurofibromas)

### ■ Other Imaging Findings

- Plain radiographs are helpful in the evaluation of spinal curvature deformities, expanded neural foramen, and scalloping.
- Computed tomography (CT): Neurofibromas are hypodense, enhancing masses. (Hypoattenuation may be related to lipid content.)
- Magnetic resonance imaging:
  - Focal areas of signal intensity (FASI)
    - Hyperintense T1 and T2 lesions (presumed hamartomas)
    - Basal ganglia, thalami, cerebellum, and subcortical white matter
    - No mass effect
    - No enhancement
  - Optic glioma
    - Optic nerve most frequently involved
    - Variable enhancement
    - Buphthalmos
- Spectroscopy can differentiate FASI from normal brain and tumors.

### ✓ Pearls & ✗ Pitfalls

- ✓ Skeletal dysplasias are the most common spinal manifestation of NF1.
- ✓ Plexiform neurofibromas can show low attenuation on noncontrasted CT scans because of the lipid content.
- ✓ Suspect NF1 in patients with dural ectasia and lateral meningoceles.
- ✓ Always study the entire neuraxis in NF1.
- ✗ Use contrast to differentiate plexiform neurofibromas from lateral meningoceles.

# Case 14

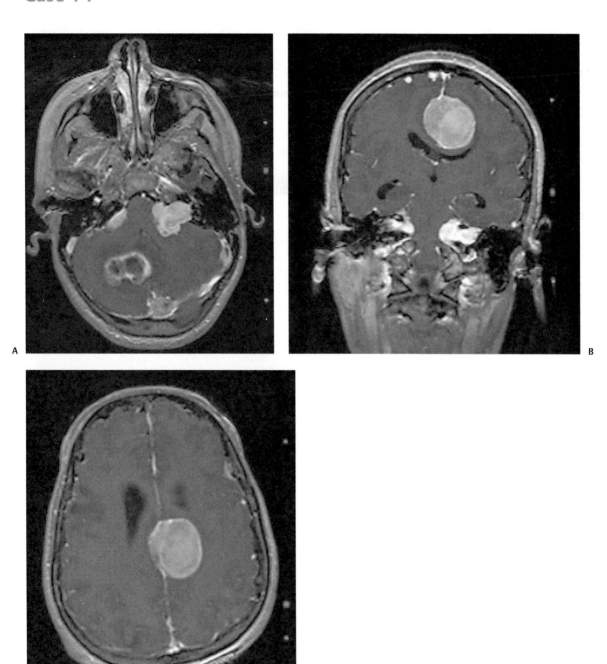

A

B

C

### ■ Clinical Presentation

A 22-year-old man presenting with hearing loss and tinnitus.

## ■ Imaging Findings

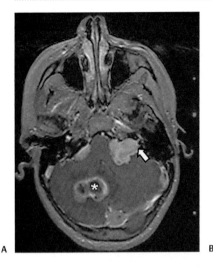
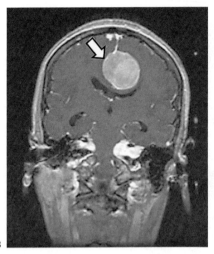
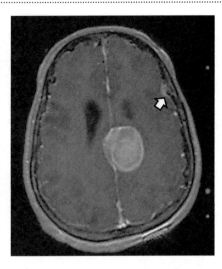

A    B    C

**(A)** Axial postcontrast image of the posterior fossa demonstrates bilateral enhancing masses in the cerebellopontine angle (CPA) cistern. On the left side, an intracanalicular component is noted (*arrow*). Two additional enhancing masses with central areas of fluid signal (*asterisk*) near the torcular and in the right cerebellum showed dural attachment in the tentorium on other images. **(B)** Coronal postcontrast image confirms the presence of CPA masses with an intracanalicular component and shows an additional enhancing lesion in the left parafalcine region with broad attachment to the dura (*arrow*). **(C)** Axial postcontrast image reveals another tiny dura-based mass in the left frontal convexity (*arrow*).

## ■ Differential Diagnosis

- **Neurofibromatosis type 2 (NF2):** Bilateral vestibular schwannomas are a defining feature of this disease. Additionally, multiple meningiomas are identified.
- *Von Hippel-Lindau syndrome:* This presents with multiple retinal and cerebellar hemangioblastomas. The lesions are parenchymal tumors, unlike the masses in the present case.
- *Dural metastasis:* Dural metastases are similar in appearance to meningiomas, but they are unusual in the CPA.

## ■ Essential Facts

- A defect in the NF2 gene on chromosome 22q11 is inherited in an autosomal-dominant fashion.
- Intracranial lesions include vestibular schwannomas (in 95% of adults, they occur in the internal auditory canal or porus acusticus); multiple meningiomas; and calcifications of the choroid plexus, cerebellar cortex, and occasionally cerebral cortex.
- Spinal lesions include cord ependymomas, multiple schwannomas of exiting nerve roots, and meningiomas.

## ■ Other Imaging Findings

- Plain radiographs are helpful in the evaluation of spinal curvature deformities, an expanded neural foramen, and scalloping.
- On computed tomography, neurofibromas appear as hypodense, enhancing masses. (Hypoattenuation may be related to lipid content.)
- Magnetic resonance imaging is excellent for the evaluation of spinal deformities and masses.

## ✓ Pearls & ✗ Pitfalls

- ✓ Cutaneous manifestations are less frequent in NF2 than in NF1; therefore, the patients are older at the time of diagnosis.
- ✓ Multiple masses along the exiting spinal nerve roots can be features of both NF1 and NF2. In NF2, these are usually schwannomas.
- ✗ Multiple tumors in a young patient should always raise suspicion for phakomatosis.

# Case 15

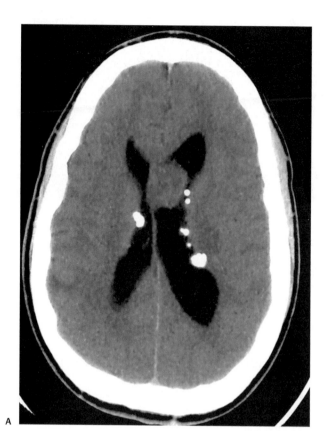

A

## Clinical Presentation

A 19-year-old man with a history of seizures presenting with progressive mental status changes.

## Further Work-up

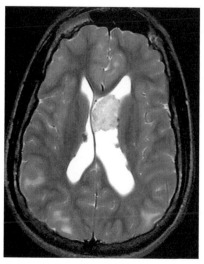

B

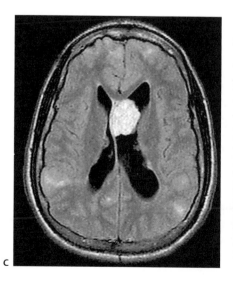

C

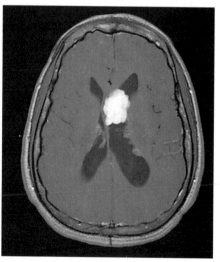

D

### ■ Imaging Findings

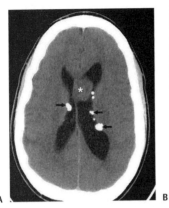
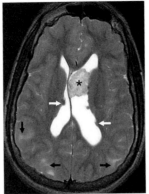
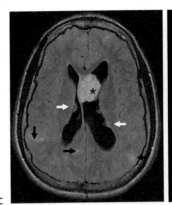
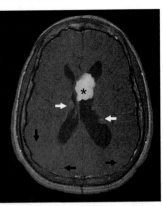

A   B   C   D

**(A)** Axial computed tomography (CT) scan of the head without contrast shows multiple subependymal calcified nodules (*arrows*). A mass is seen in the left lateral ventricle adjacent to the septum pellucidum (*asterisk*). Note the dilatation of the left ventricle due to obstruction of the foramen of Monro on that side. **(B)** Axial T2-weighted image (WI) of the brain shows multiple subependymal nodules (*white arrows*). A giant cell astrocytoma with heterogeneous signal (*asterisk*) is deforming the septum pellucidum. Multiple subcortical and cortical tubers are seen as areas of hyperintensity (*black arrows*). **(C)** Fluid-attenuated inversion recovery (FLAIR) image of the brain shows multiple subependymal nodules (*white arrows*). A giant cell astrocytoma with heterogeneous signal (*asterisk*) is deforming the septum pellucidum. Multiple subcortical and cortical tubers are seen as areas of hyperintensity (*black arrows*). **(D)** Axial T1-weighted postcontrast magnetic resonance imaging (MRI) of the brain shows multiple enhancing subependymal nodules (*white arrows*). An enhancing giant cell astrocytoma (*asterisk*) is displacing the septum pellucidum on the right. Multiple subcortical and cortical tubers do not show enhancement (*black arrows*).

### ■ Differential Diagnosis

- **Tuberous sclerosis complex (Bourneville-Pringle syndrome):** In this diagnosis, look for cortical and subcortical tubers, subependymal nodules, subependymal giant cell astrocytomas, and white matter radial migration lines (heterotopic glia).
- *Central neurocytoma:* Central neurocytoma is in the differential diagnosis for a frontal intraventricular mass. This tumor consists of a well-circumscribed mass that is confined to the anterior portion of the lateral ventricles. No subependymal nodules or cortical tubers are present. There are punctate calcifications within the mass. Multiple small cysts can be seen. There is mild to moderate contrast enhancement. Central neurocytomas rarely extend outside the ventricles.
- *Congenital cytomegalovirus infection:* Periventricular and parenchymal calcifications are seen in congenital cytomegalovirus infection, as are microcephaly, cortical gyral abnormalities (agyria and thin cortex), hippocampal dysplasia, and cerebellar hypoplasia.

### ■ Essential Facts

- Tuberous sclerosis complex is a phakomatosis caused by abnormal differentiation of the cells of the germinal matrix and is associated with migrational neuronal arrest.
- Cortical and subcortical tubers are dysmorphic neurons. Ninety percent are cerebral and 10% are cerebellar. Only 3% enhance.
- Subependymal nodules are seen in the walls of the lateral ventricles. They calcify and may enhance. Malignant degeneration to giant cell astrocytoma occurs in 10 to 15%.

- Microcephaly is usually present as a consequence of brain volume loss.
- Tuberous sclerosis is associated with rhabdomyoma of the heart, angiomyolipomas of the kidneys (50%), drusen, and cystic lesions.

### ■ Other Imaging Findings

- Computed tomography can demonstrate calcification in the subependymal nodules and ventriculomegaly.
- On MRI, cortical and subcortical tubers appear as areas of high signal on T2WIs and FLAIR images.
- Positron emission tomography can identify epileptogenic tubers (tubers that are disproportionately hypometabolic for their size).

### ✓ Pearls & ✗ Pitfalls

- ✓ Tubers are multiple in 95% of patients.
- ✓ Ninety percent of tubers are located in the frontal lobes.
- ✗ In newborns, the nodular subependymal lesions appear hyperintense on T1WIs and hypointense on T2WIs (the reverse of what is seen in adults) because of the lack of myelination.

# Case 16

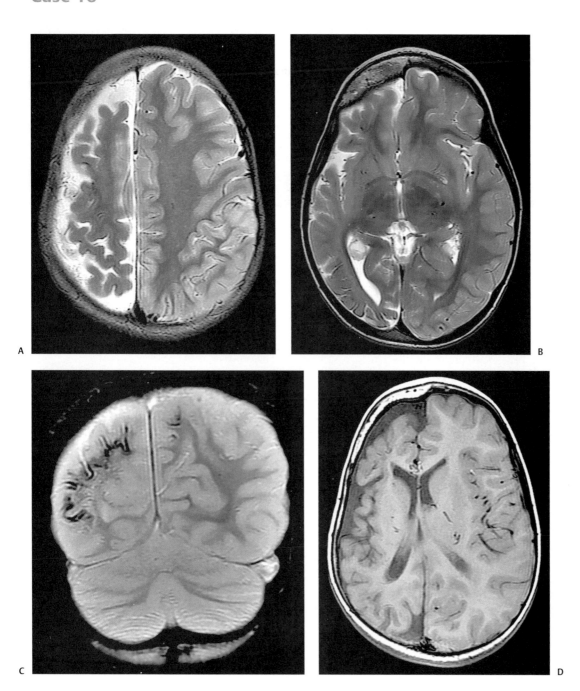

## Clinical Presentation

A 17-year-old girl with seizures, hemiparesis, and homonymous hemianopsia.

## ■ Imaging Findings

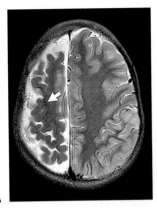
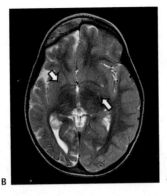
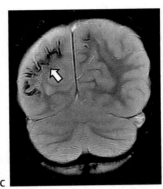
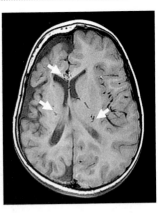

A    B    C    D

**(A)** Axial T2-weighted image (WI) of the brain demonstrates atrophy of the right cerebral hemisphere and linear areas of decreased signal along the cortex (*arrow*). **(B)** Axial T2WI of the brain demonstrates atrophy of the right cerebral hemisphere. Flow voids of dilated ependymal veins are also noted (*arrows*). **(C)** Coronal gradient-echo image reveals tram-track cortical calcifications in the atrophic right hemisphere (*arrow*). Less extensive changes are present in the left parietal cortex. **(D)** Note the dilated medullary veins, which appear as large flow voids on the axial T1WI (*arrows*).

## ■ Differential Diagnosis

- **Sturge-Weber syndrome (also known as encephalotrigeminal angiomatosis):** There is atrophy of the affected hemisphere with tram-track cortical calcifications. The calvarium is thickened.
- *Cortical laminar necrosis from old hemispheric infarct:* More significant volume loss and dilatation of the ventricles would be expected in this diagnosis. Dilatation of the medullary and subependymal veins is not a feature of cortical laminar necrosis.
- *Superficial siderosis:* Hemosiderin is deposited along the leptomeninges, subpial tissues, and subependyma of the ventricles as a result of chronic, recurrent subarachnoid hemorrhage. T2-weighted and gradient-echo images reveal hypointensity along the pial surface of the brain and spinal cord and along the ependyma of the ventricles.

## ■ Essential Facts

- The postcapillary circulation of the brain and face is abnormal.
- A facial port wine stain and choroidal, scleral, or episcleral telangiectasia are characteristic.
- Abnormal venous drainage of the hemispheres results in the recruitment of collateral veins from the choroid plexus and medullary veins.
- Chronic cerebral ischemia leads to atrophy and calcification.

## ■ Other Imaging Findings

- On computed tomography (CT), tram-track calcification is unusual before 2 years of age.
- Magnetic resonance imaging shows contrast enhancement of the subarachnoid space, calcifications on T2- and T2*WIs, enlargement of the choroid plexi, and T2 prolongation in the adjacent white matter.
- Functional neuroimaging with fluorodeoxyglucose positron emission tomography often demonstrates cortical hypometabolism extending beyond the apparent structural abnormalities in Sturge-Weber syndrome.

## ✓ Pearls & ✗ Pitfalls

- ✓ The Dyke-Davidoff-Masson sequence consists of unilateral skull and sinus hypertrophy (mainly the frontal sinus), then atrophy of the mastoid air cells and ipsilateral cerebral hemisphere (in childhood). Causes are cerebral infarction (most often), infection, trauma, and Sturge-Weber syndrome.
- ✗ Tram-track calcifications of the brain may mask contrast enhancement on CT.

# Case 17

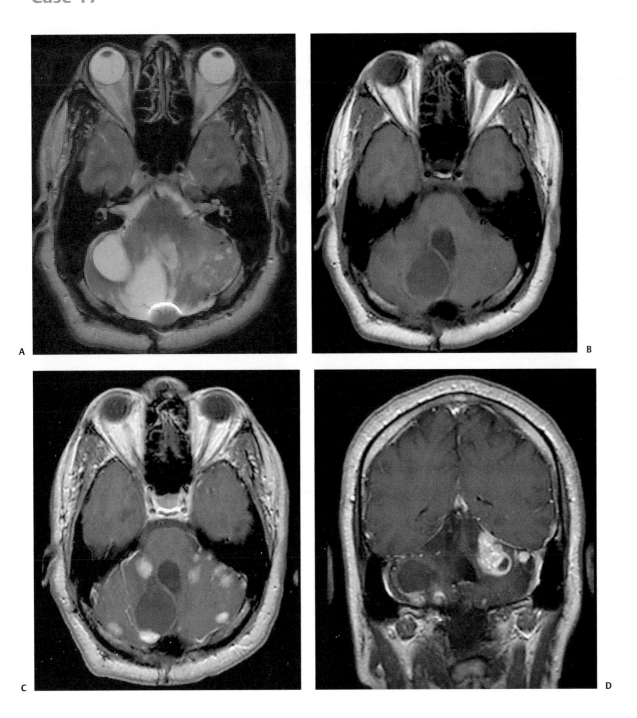

## ■ Clinical Presentation

A 35-year-old man with the history of a resected tumor in the cerebellum presenting with worsening dysmetria.

### ■ Imaging Findings

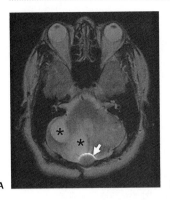
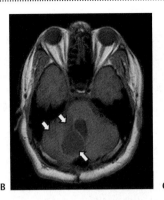
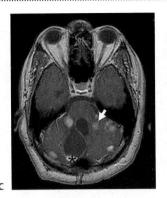
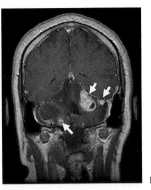

A    B    C    D

**(A)** Axial T2-weighted image (WI) demonstrates multiple cystic lesions (*asterisks*) in the cerebellum bilaterally and areas of encephalomalacia on the left side. Note the magnetic susceptibility artifact near the occipital bone resulting from prior surgery (*arrow*). **(B)** Axial T1WI of the brain without contrast showing well-defined cystic lesions with signal slightly higher than that of cerebrospinal fluid (*arrows*). **(C)** Axial postcontrast T1WI shows numerous enhancing solid lesions (*arrow*) and a mural nodule (*asterisk*) along the wall of one of the cerebellar cysts. **(D)** Coronal postcontrast T1WI shows numerous enhancing solid lesions (*arrows*) and a mural nodule (*asterisk*) along the wall of one of the cerebellar cysts.

### ■ Differential Diagnosis

- ***Von Hippel-Lindau (VHL) disease (also known as hemangioblastomatosis):*** Multiple hemangioblastomas in the posterior fossa, which are cystic with a mural nodule, are characteristic of this diagnosis. No surrounding vasogenic edema is present.
- *Metastatic disease:* this presents as numerous mass lesions with surrounding edema and mass effect.
- *Multiple brain abscesses:* These are characterized by multiple necrotic, thick, ring-enhancing lesions with significant edema and without a mural nodule. It is unusual for only the cerebellum to be involved.

### ■ Essential Facts

- The VHL gene on chromosome 3 is inherited in an autosomal-dominant fashion.
- Central nervous system (CNS) neoplasms include hemangioblastomas in the cerebellum, brainstem, spinal cord, and retina as well as endolymphatic sac tumors.
- Non-CNS lesions include clear cell renal carcinoma, pheochromocytoma, pancreatic neuroendocrine tumors, and epididymal cystadenoma.
- Hemangioblastomas are solid, cystic, hemorrhagic, or mixed. They are frequently cystic with a mural enhancing nodule.
- Hemangioblastomas may have flow voids from feeding arteries.

### ■ Other Imaging Findings

- Hemangioblastomas are highly vascular lesions, demonstrating arterial blush on conventional angiography. There is no arteriovenous shunting.

### ✓ Pearls & ✗ Pitfalls

- ✓ Hemangioblastomas may occur sporadically; however, 20 to 38% of cerebellar hemangioblastomas are associated with VHL disease.
- ✓ Spinal hemangioblastomas are infrequent and highly suggestive of VHL disease.
- ✗ Spinal cord hemangioblastomas may be mistaken for drop metastases from a cerebellar hemangioblastoma.

# Case 18

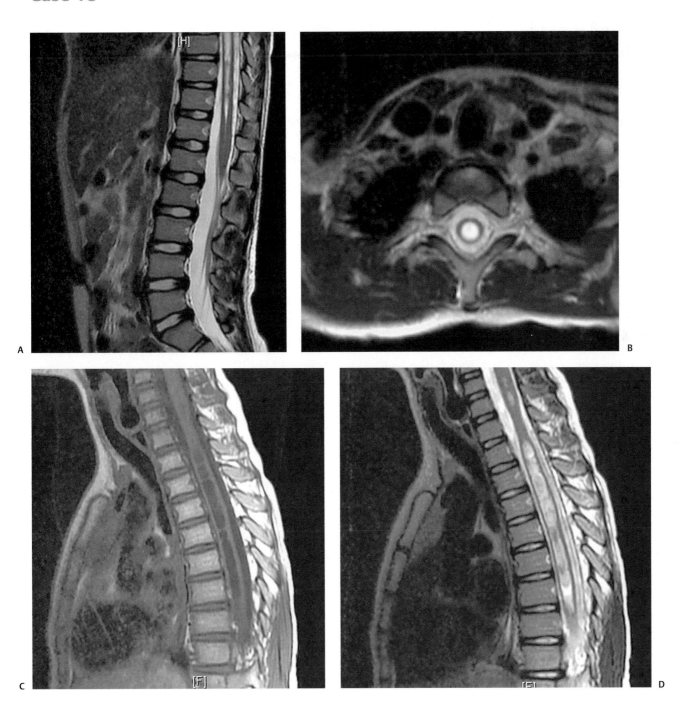

## Clinical Presentation

A 7-year-old boy with neck paresthesias and hand tingling.

## ■ Imaging Findings

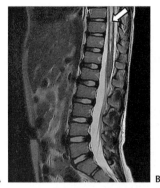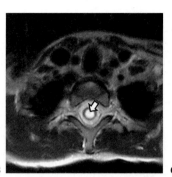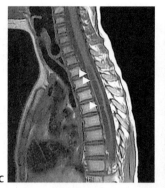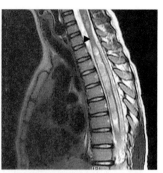

A     B     C     D

**(A)** Sagittal T2-weighted image (WI) of the lower spine demonstrates a well-defined central area of fluid signal within the cord, which tapers toward the conus medullaris (*arrow*). **(B)** Axial T2WI in the cervical region shows a central fluid cavity within the cord with well-defined margins (*arrow*). There is mild cord expansion. **(C)** Sagittal T1WI shows extension of the cystic cavity to the cervical cord and multiple septa (*arrowheads*). **(D)** Sagittal T2WI of the upper spine demonstrates expansion of the cord in the area that contains the fluid cavity, with a waist in the region where the cord is normal (*arrowhead*).

## ■ Differential Diagnosis

- **Syringohydromyelia:** This is characterized by a longitudinally oriented cavity within the spinal cord, with cerebrospinal fluid (CSF) signal on all the sequences. There is no solid component or enhancement.
- *Myelomalacia:* Myelomalacia has moderately increased T2 signal and moderately reduced T1 signal relative to the cord, poorly defined margins, and no CSF flow artifacts.
- *Cystic astrocytoma:* Cystic astrocytoma is an eccentrically located lesion with low T1 signal and high T2 signal relative to the cord. It has a cystic component in 25 to 38% of cases. If the cystic component is lined with tumor cells, it usually demonstrates peripheral wall enhancement, unlike a secondary syrinx.

## ■ Essential Facts

- A longitudinally oriented, fluid-filled cavity originates in the spinal cord tissue or in the central canal.
- Distinguishing between hydromyelia (dilatation of the central canal) and syringomyelia (the cavity is lateral to the central canal) is frequently not possible.
- Causes may be congenital, tumor-related (astrocytoma, glioma, ependymoma), trauma-related, or infective/inflammatory.

## ■ Other Imaging Findings

- Magnetic resonance imaging shows single or multiple cystic intramedullary collections with CSF signal on all sequences, tapered cranial and caudal ends, and expansion of the cord. The lesion may have a beaded appearance.
- Atypical signal: The T1 signal is high when the lesion contains infected or proteinaceous material. An artifactual low T2 signal is due to CSF pulsation.

## ✓ Pearls & ✗ Pitfalls

- ✓ When a syrinx is initially found on imaging, the full craniocaudal extent needs to be assessed. If no obvious cause is identified, gadolinium-enhanced images must be obtained in an attempt to detect any underlying tumor.
- ✓ Syrinx cavities that are secondary to Chiari malformations, foramen magnum stenosis, or tumor may resolve after blockage of the CSF circulation is resolved.
- ✗ Gibbs or truncation artifacts are bright or dark lines that are seen parallel and adjacent to the borders of abrupt changes in intensity, such as the transition from bright CSF to dark spinal cord on a T2WI. In the spinal cord, this artifact can simulate a small syrinx to the unaware.
- ✗ Ventriculus terminalis is a nonenhancing, ovoid, nonseptate cystic structure localized within a normally positioned conus; it is seen frequently in patients younger than 5 years of age.

# Case 19

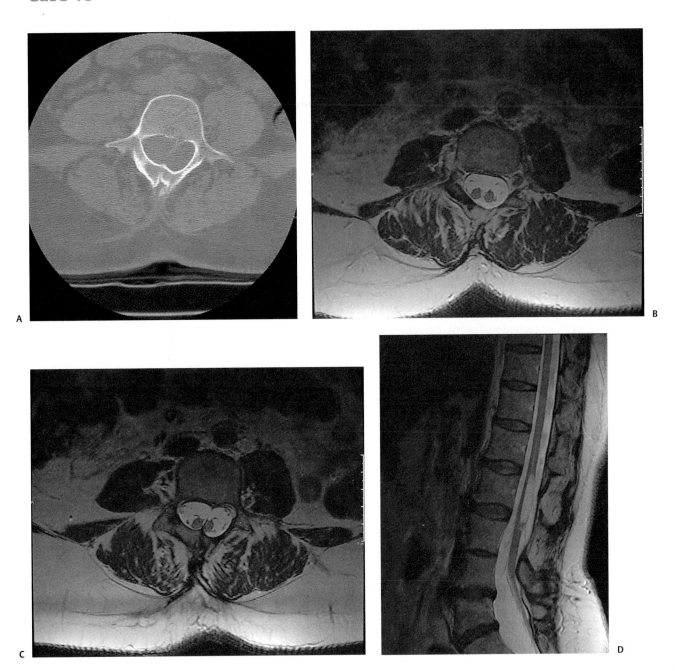

## Clinical Presentation

A 40-year-old woman with progressive leg weakness that has worsened in the last year.

## ■ Imaging Findings

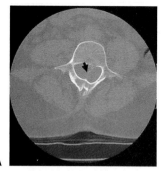
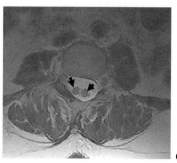
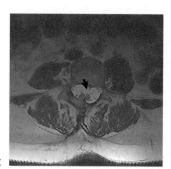
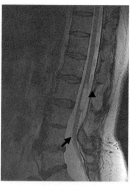

**(A)** Axial computed tomography (CT) scan of the lumbar spine demonstrates a bony spur in the spinal canal (*arrow*). **(B)** Axial T2-weighted image (WI) of the lumbar spine shows two hemicords (*arrows*) inside the thecal sac. **(C)** Axial T2-weighted magnetic resonance imaging (MRI) of the lumbar spine demonstrates the septum (*arrow*) dividing the spinal cord. **(D)** Sagittal T2WI of the lumbar spine shows a tethered cord. The cystlike lesion (*arrow*) is where the cord splits (*arrowhead*).

## ■ Differential Diagnosis

- ***Diastematomyelia (split cord malformation):*** Diastematomyelia is a focal or complete split of the spinal cord. It is the consequence of a split notochord. It is associated with congenital scoliosis (80% of cases), tethered cord syndrome (75% of cases), and spinal bony anomalies (50% of cases). Intersegmental laminar fusion is pathognomonic.
- *Meningocele manqué:* Meningocele manqué is characterized by dysraphic dorsal tethered bands (atretic neural tissue) adherent to dura. The following may be seen: diastematomyelia, filum lipoma, dermoid cysts, and neuroenteric cysts. These are difficult to see on imaging studies.
- *Tethered cord syndrome:* Tethered cord syndrome is characterized by a low-lying conus medullaris (below L2; some authors say below L3). Traction of the spinal cord is secondary to closed spinal dysraphism, diastematomyelia, spinal lipoma, tight filum terminale, caudal regression syndrome, scar tissue after meningocele repair, thickened filum terminale, and hydromyelia, and it is associated with progressive neurologic deterioration.

## ■ Essential Facts

- There are two types of diastematomyelia:
  - Type 1 (with septum): 25%
    ○ A bony septum results in separate dural tubes, each containing a hemicord.
    ○ The usual location is the thoracic or lumbar spine.
    ○ Scoliosis is present.
    ○ Hydromyelia is common.
  - Type 2 (without septum): 75%
    ○ There is no bony spur; a fibrous septum may be present.
    ○ Only one thecal sac contains both hemicords.

## ■ Other Imaging Findings

- Plain radiographs are limited but can detect scoliosis and vertebral anomalies.
- CT can demonstrate the bony spur and hemivertebrae.
- Myelo-CT is a helpful tool to demonstrate the dural sac and hemicords.
- MRI:
  - Axial and coronal views are best to demonstrate the split cord. This is difficult to see on sagittal images.
  - T2 is best to demonstrate hydrosyringomyelia.
  - It is limited in the evaluation of a bony spur.
  - It can demonstrate a dermal sinus.

## ✓ Pearls & ✗ Pitfalls

- ✓ Cutaneous birthmarks (hemangiomas, dyschromic patches, and hairy tufts) overlie the defect in 50% of cases.
- ✓ Females are more often affected than males.
- ✓ Intersegmental laminar fusion is pathognomonic.
- ✓ Image the spine of a patient whose skin marks are compatible with the cutaneous stigmata of diastematomyelia.
- ✗ Diastematomyelia is very hard to see in sagittal views.
- ✗ Evaluation for a bony spur is limited in MRI.
- ✗ Meningocele manqué is hardly ever diagnosed with imaging (it is diagnosed surgically).

# Case 20

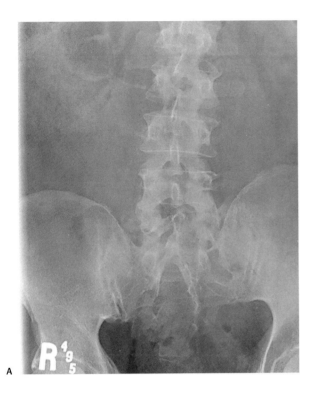

A

## Clinical Presentation

A patient with urinary incontinence and a subcutaneous mass in the sacral region.

## Further Work-up

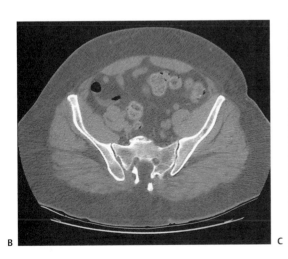

B

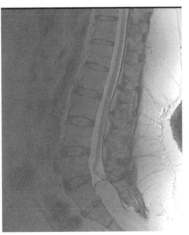

C

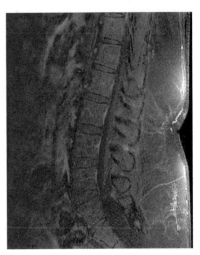

D

## ■ Imaging Findings

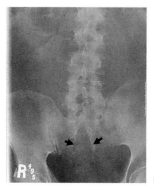
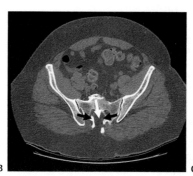
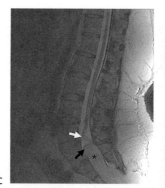
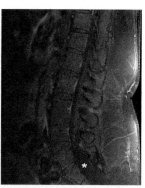

**(A)** Anteroposterior radiograph of the lumbar spine shows dysraphism of the sacrum (*arrows*). **(B)** Axial computed tomography (CT) scan of the pelvis without contrast demonstrates the lack of fusion of the posterior elements of the sacrum (*black arrows*). Fat corresponding to the lipoma occupies the defect (*white arrow*). **(C)** Sagittal T2-weighted image (WI) of the lumbar spine shows the conus descending to L4 (*white arrow*). The lipoma extends into the spinal canal (*asterisk*). The *black arrow* points to the placode-lipoma interface. **(D)** Sagittal T1WI of the lumbar spine with fat saturation and contrast; note the fat suppression of the lipoma (*asterisk*).

## ■ Differential Diagnosis

- **Lipomyelocele and lipomyelomeningocele:** Lipomyeloceles and lipomyelomeningoceles are large subcutaneous lipomas with intraspinal extension through a wide spina bifida. Tethered cord is present in all cases. Skin abnormalities can occur in 50% of the cases: hypertrichosis, dimple, dermal sinus tract, and capillary hemangioma.
- *Myelomeningocele (dorsal):* This is a less extensive spinal dysraphism. Dermal stigmata or a mass can be present, but no lipoma is associated. Myelomeningocele is not always associated with tethered cord.
- *Sacrococcygeal teratoma:* This is a complex pelvic mass in newborns characterized by fat, calcifications in 60% of cases, debris, skin appendages, and enhancement of the solid portions.

## ■ Essential Facts

- This is an abnormality of primary neurulation.
- The junction between fat and meninges is intact in lipomyelocele and lipomyelomeningocele.
- Lipomyelocele, also known as lipomyeloschisis (75% of cases): the placode-lipoma interface is inside the spinal canal.
- Lipomyelomeningocele (25% of cases): the placode-lipoma interface is outside the spinal canal in a meningocele.
- Plain radiography demonstrates sacral dysraphism.
- On CT, fat occupies the spinal canal, and bony defects are identified.
- T2WIs can detect the placode-lipoma interface; fat-saturated sequences confirm the lipoma.
- There is no enhancement.

## ■ Other Imaging Findings

- Obstetric ultrasound can show posterior dysraphism and fat in the lipomatous portion.

## ✓ Pearls & ✗ Pitfalls

- ✓ Because of its origin, the lipomatous portion of the lesion is extradural in location.
- ✓ The lipoma is asymmetric in almost half of the cases.
- ✓ If a dorsal myelomeningocele is associated with a tethered cord, look for a lipoma.
- ✗ Meningoceles are associated in only 25% of cases (lipomyelomeningocele).

# Case 21

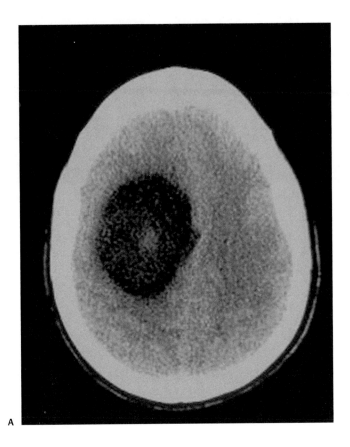

A

## ▪ Clinical Presentation

A 25-year-old woman presenting with headaches and papilledema.

## Further Work-up

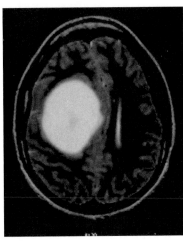

B

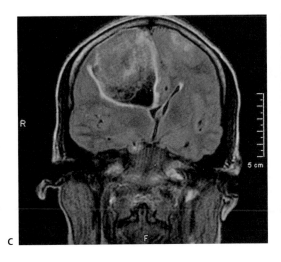

C

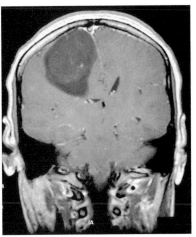

D

### ■ Imaging Findings

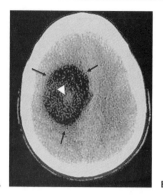
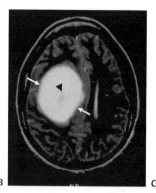
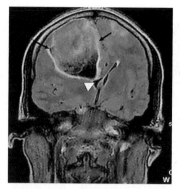
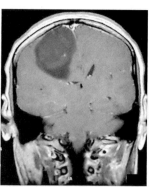

A   B   C   D

**(A)** Computed tomography (CT) scan without contrast shows a round, hypoattenuated lesion in the right frontal lobe (*arrows*). The lesion is located in the subcortical white matter and demonstrates a coarse central calcification (*arrowhead*). **(B)** Axial T2-weighted image (WI) shows a hyperintense subcortical mass (*arrows*) in the right frontal lobe; no vasogenic edema is evident. An area of low signal is seen in the center of the mass (*arrowhead*), representing the calcification evident on the CT scan. **(C)** Coronal fluid-attenuated inversion recovery image shows a mass in the right frontal lobe with heterogeneous signal (*arrows*). There is effacement of the right frontal horn (*arrowhead*) and displacement of the midline to the left. **(D)** Coronal T1WI with contrast shows mild enhancement of the right frontal mass.

### ■ Differential Diagnosis

- **Oligodendroglioma:** This is a tumor of glial origin presenting as a mass in the cortex or subcortical white matter with coarse calcification (20–90% of cases) and occasional cystic degeneration or hemorrhage. Most do not enhance, but there may be subtle enhancement in 20%. They are more frequently supratentorial in location (90% of cases). Vasogenic edema is uncommon.
- *Low-grade astrocytoma:* In low-grade astrocytoma, the location is more central, and the cortex is rarely involved. Calcification is infrequent. All the other characteristics are similar to those of oligodendroglioma.
- *Dysembryoplastic neuroepithelial tumor (DNET):* DNET is a benign, well-marginated lesion. DNET has a cortical location but is more frequently in the temporal lobe. It has a "bubbly" appearance on magnetic resonance imaging (MRI), variable enhancement (20%), and calcification (25%). It presents in patients younger than 20 years of age, usually with seizures.

### ■ Essential Facts

- Calcification is associated with higher-grade tumors.
- Calcification and vasogenic edema are rare in children.
- Low-grade tumors (World Health Organization [WHO] grades I and II) are called oligodendrogliomas.
- High-grade oligodendrogliomas (WHO grade III) are called anaplastic oligodendrogliomas.

### ■ Other Imaging Findings

- CT: Sixty percent have low attenuation and 23% are isodense to the parenchyma. DNETs may not be detected on CT.
- MRI:
  - Better definition of tumor extent
  - Typically heterogeneous signal
  - T1WIs: hypointense to gray matter
  - T2WIs: hyperintense to gray matter
  - Diffusion-WIs: higher-grade tumors tend to have lower apparent diffusion coefficient values.

### ✓ Pearls & ✗ Pitfalls

- ✓ Tumors with 1p and 19q deletions are more likely to calcify and have ill-defined margins; even though these tumors tend to be more aggressive, they also respond better to chemotherapy.
- ✓ The more aggressive variant—anaplastic oligodendroglioma (WHO grade III)—is commonly associated with these deletions.
- ✓ Consider DNET if a cortically based tumor in the temporal lobe presents in a young patient.
- ✗ Oligodendrogliomas are the most common intracranial tumors that have calcifications; however, only 20% calcify.

# Case 22

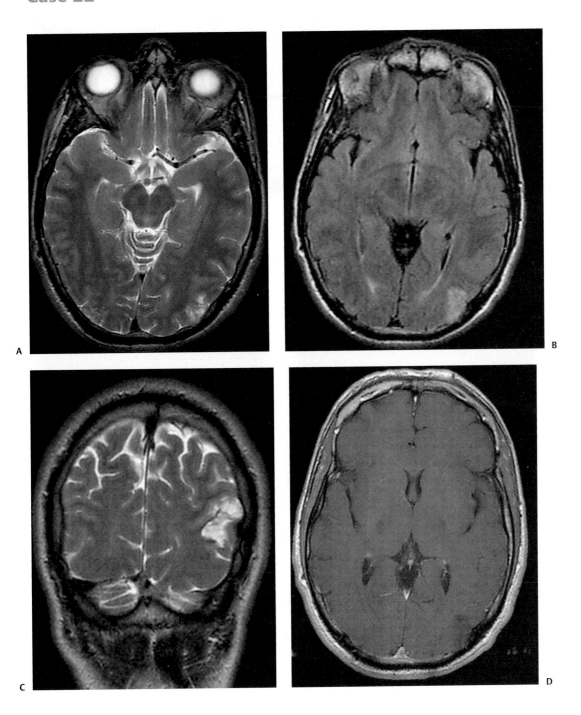

## Clinical Presentation

A 27-year-old with a history of seizures.

■ **Imaging Findings**

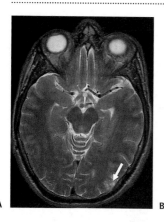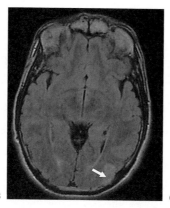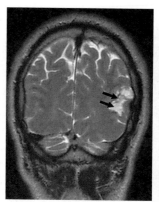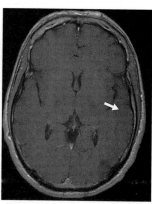

A    B    C    D

**(A)** Axial T2-weighted image (WI) of the brain shows a lesion in the left parietal lobe (*arrow*) with a small, cystic, "bubbly" appearance. **(B)** Axial fluid-attenuated inversion recovery (FLAIR) image demonstrates increased cortical signal in the left parietal lobe (*arrow*) without surrounding edema. **(C)** Coronal T2WI demonstrates the cortically based, "bubbly" lesion (*arrows*) in the left parietal lobe. **(D)** Axial T1WI with contrast shows no enhancement in the left parietal mass (*arrow*).

■ **Differential Diagnosis**

• *Dysembryoplastic neuroepithelial tumor (DNET):* DNETs are benign, well-demarcated cortical lesions. They present as partial seizures in patients younger than 20 years. They occur more frequently in the temporal lobe (60%) or frontal lobe (30%). Cortical dysplasia is often noted adjacent to the lesion. Calcification is rare (20%). DNET appears as a multilobulated "bubbly" lesion with high signal on T2WIs and low signal on T1WIs. There is no surrounding vasogenic edema. Thirty percent show enhancement.
• *Ganglioglioma:* Ganglioglioma is also a mixed neuronal glial cell tumor. This is a cystic mass and does not have the multilobulated appearance of DNET. Ganglioglioma presents as a mural enhancing nodule (40%), has a temporal lobe distribution, and is calcified in 30% of cases. It can scallop the inner table of the skull. There is no associated vasogenic edema.
• *Neuroepithelial cyst:* Neuroepithelial cysts are thin-walled and can be uni- or multilocular. They have no enhancement. The intraventricular location is more common. They do not have a bright rim on FLAIR images.

■ **Essential Facts**

• Initially described in 1988
• Mixed neuronal glial cell tumor
• Located in the temporal lobe, usually near the amygdala of the hippocampus
• Inner scalloping of the skull

■ **Other Imaging Findings**

• Computed tomography (CT): Low density. CT can detect the calcifications, even though they are rare. CT allows the evaluation of inner table scalloping.
• Magnetic resonance imaging: faint enhancement (20%) and a bright rim are seen on FLAIR images.

✓ **Pearls & ✗ Pitfalls**

✓ Look for a FLAIR rim.
✓ The multilobulated morphology helps in the differential diagnosis.
✓ Exclude DNET from your differential list in adult patients.
✗ On CT, DNET can resemble a stroke; however, it does not evolve to secondary atrophy.

# Case 23

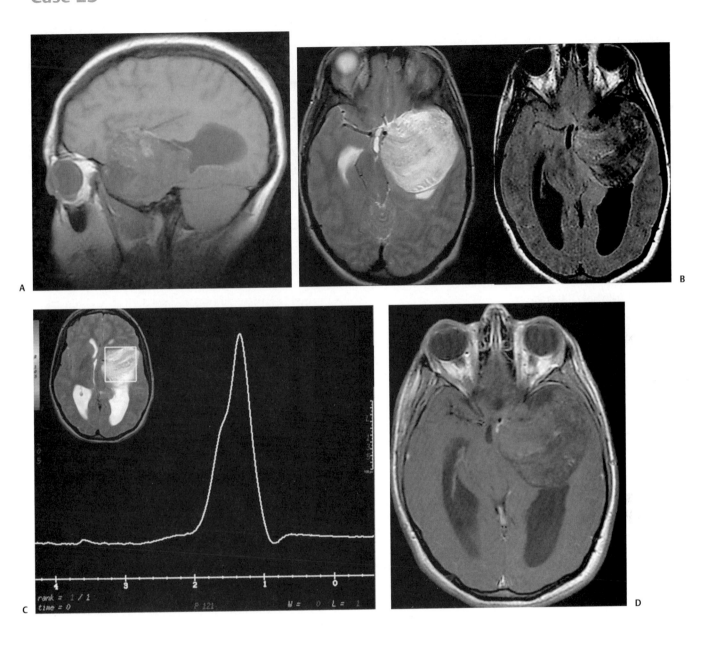

A

B

C

D

## Clinical Presentation

A 17-year-old girl with a history of seizures.

## ■ Imaging Findings

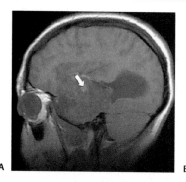
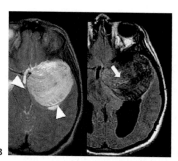
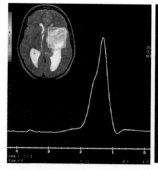
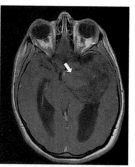

**(A)** Sagittal T1-weighted image (WI) shows a mass in the anterior aspect of the temporal fossa with areas of T1 hyperintensity (*arrow*). The mass is compressing the adjacent parenchyma. **(B)** Axial T2-weighted and fluid-attenuated inversion recovery (FLAIR) images demonstrate heterogeneous signal in the left temporal fossa mass. The mass shows areas of increased signal on the FLAIR image (*arrow*). The location of the lesion is extra-axial. It compresses the temporal lobe and cerebellar peduncle (*arrowheads*), displacing vessels without encasing them. **(C)** Magnetic resonance (MR) spectroscopy shows a high lipid peak with a broad base from −0.9 to −1.3 parts per million (ppm). **(D)** Axial T1WI with contrast shows no enhancement of the mass; the hyperintense regions (*arrow*) were bright in the nonenhanced sequences (related to fat).

## ■ Differential Diagnosis

- **Nonruptured dermoid cyst:** Dermoid cysts are ectodermal inclusion cysts that contain squamous and glandular tissue. The tissue causes the cysts to grow, increasing the likelihood of ruptures. They account for fewer than 5% of intracranial tumors and are most frequent in the midline. A supratentorial location is more common than an infratentorial location. If a cyst ruptures, chemical meningitis develops with secondary vasospasm and stroke; the contents can be intraventricular. They have a well-defined capsule that is thicker than the capsule in epidermoid cysts.
- *Epidermoid cyst:* Epidermoid cysts are also ectodermal inclusion cysts, although they contain only squamous epithelium. The signal characteristics are similar to those of cerebrospinal fluid (CSF), except for slight hyperintensity and heterogeneity on FLAIR images ("dirty CSF appearance"). They are five to nine times more common than dermoid cysts. They are less common in pediatric patients. The most frequent locations are around the cerebellopontine angle and the ventricles. They typically show restricted diffusion and no contrast enhancement.
- *Craniopharyngioma:* Craniopharyngiomas are benign dysontogenetic epithelial masses that originate at the epithelium of the Rathke pouch. They are the most common pediatric tumors in the suprasellar region. They have mixed solid and cystic components with calcification. Most of them enhance (90%). Calcifications can be seen on computed tomography or gradient-echo T2*WIs. Cyst contents are typically hyperintense on FLAIR images.

## ■ Essential Facts

- The sellar, parasellar, and frontonasal regions are common locations for nonruptured dermoid cysts.

- Dermoid cysts contain ectodermal derivatives such as squamous epithelium and dermal appendages such as hair follicles, sebaceous glands, and apocrine glands, which produce keratin and oils.
- The meninges enhance when rupture and chemical meningitis have occurred; otherwise, no enhancement is noted.

## ■ Other Imaging Findings

- Computed tomography:
  - Round, lobulated mass with low attenuation (cholesterol content)
    - Capsular calcification in 20%
    - Can remodel the adjacent skull
- MR imaging: hyperintense on T1; both hypo- and hyperintense regions common on T2
  - If ruptured: typical appearance of fat-fluid levels in the frontal horns; diffuse, hyperintense droplets in the subarachnoid or intraventricular spaces on T1WIs; extensive pial enhancement on T1WIs with contrast
  - Broad lipid peak on MR spectroscopy

## ✓ Pearls & ✗ Pitfalls

- ✓ Both dermoid and epidermoid cysts are ectodermal inclusion cysts; the difference is that dermoid cysts contain squamous epithelium and skin appendages, whereas epidermoid cysts are lined only by squamous epithelium.
- ✓ Ruptured and unruptured dermoid cysts differ in appearance.
- ✓ Enhancement is rarely seen and is usually secondary to chemical meningitis.

# Case 24

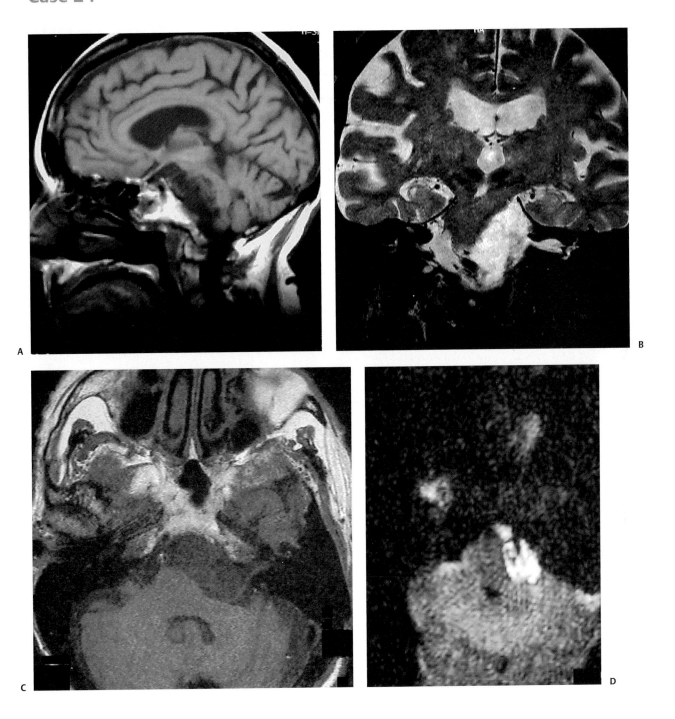

## Clinical Presentation

A 35-year-old man with progressive left-sided hearing loss.

### ■ Imaging Findings

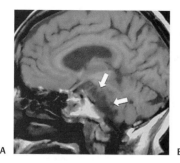 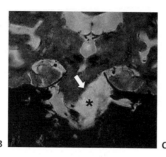 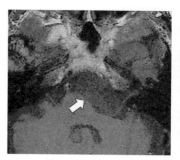 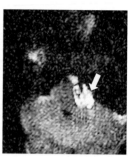

**(A)** Sagittal T1-weighted image (WI) shows the irregular anterior border of the pons (*arrows*). **(B)** Coronal T2WI demonstrates displacement of the pons to the right (*arrow*). A lesion in the left cerebellopontine angle (CPA) has a slightly higher signal than that of cerebrospinal fluid (CSF; *asterisk*). **(C)** Axial T1WI shows a lesion in the left CPA that has a signal like that of CSF and displaces the pons to the right (*arrow*). **(D)** Diffusion-WI demonstrates high signal in the mass located in the left CPA (*arrow*).

### ■ Differential Diagnosis

- **Epidermoid cyst:** Ectodermal inclusion cysts are composed of epithelial cells that form a keratohyalin matrix as a consequence of desquamation. The location is usually away from the midline in the basal subarachnoid cisterns and ventricles. The cysts engulf vessel and nerves. Epidermoid cysts have a signal like that of CSF on T1 and T2WIs but have a heterogeneous signal on fluid-attenuated inversion recovery (FLAIR) images. They have a high signal on diffusion-WIs secondary to T2 "shine through." They do not enhance.
- **Dermoid cyst:** Dermoid cysts are also ectodermal inclusion cysts that, in addition to squamous epithelium, contain skin appendages that form cholesterol. They have a heterogeneous signal, with areas of high T1 signal secondary to fatty content. They tend to have a midline location. Dermoid cysts can rupture and cause chemical meningitis. Typically, there is no enhancement, although the meninges may enhance if the cysts rupture. A supratentorial location is more common. Dermoid cysts do not have a signal on diffusion-WIs.
- **Arachnoid cyst:** These are CSF-filled cysts. They have a signal like that of CSF in all sequences. There is no signal on diffusion-WIs. There is no enhancement. The middle cranial fossa is the most common location (50%), followed by the CPA (10%). Arachnoid cysts displace cortical vessels away from the calvarium.

### ■ Essential Facts

- The CPA is most common location for epidermoid cysts (45%), followed by the 4th ventricle (15%).
- The lesion encases arteries without compromising the lumina.
- On computed tomography, they resemble CSF and rarely calcify (20%).
- On magnetic resonance imaging, the lesions are isointense to CSF on T1WIs and slightly hyperintense to CSF on T2WIs. On FLAIR images, they show a signal slightly higher than that of CSF. On diffusion-WIs, they show T2 "shine through."

### ✓ Pearls & ✗ Pitfalls

- ✓ Very rare degeneration to squamous cell carcinoma has been seen.
- ✓ Dermoid cysts are more common in the supratentorial territory, whereas epidermoid cysts are more frequent in the infratentorial region.
- ✗ The high signal of epidermoid cysts on diffusion-WIs is caused by T2 "shine through," not restricted diffusion.
- ✗ Rare cases of epidermoid cysts with a high protein content have been reported as hyperdense with a high signal on T1 and T2WIs.

# Case 25

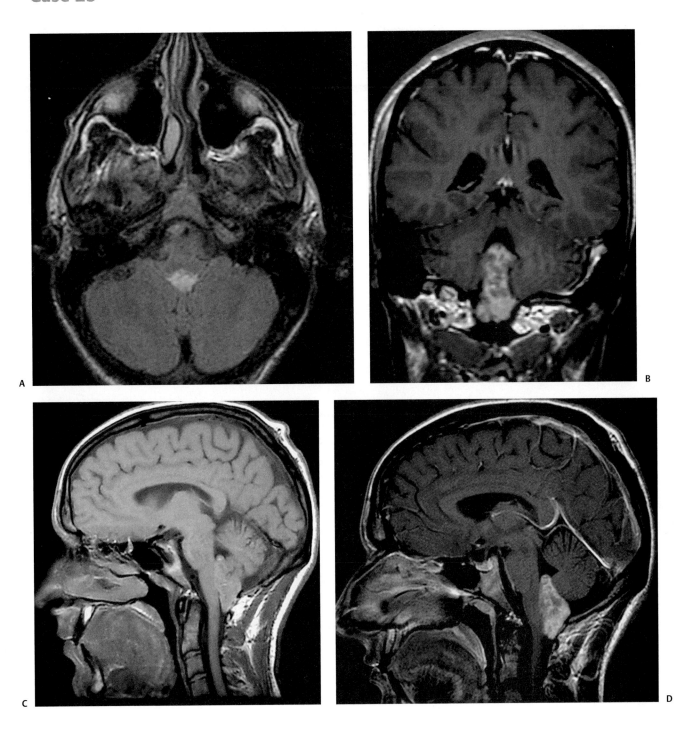

A

B

C

D

## ▨ Clinical Presentation

A 28-year-old man presenting with ataxia, headache, nausea, and vomiting.

## Imaging Findings

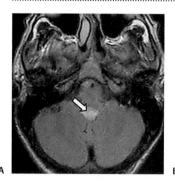
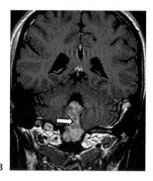
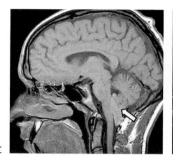
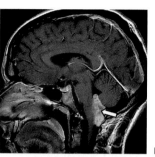

A          B          C          D

**(A)** Axial fluid-attenuated inversion recovery (FLAIR) image shows a well-defined hyperdense lesion occupying the 4th ventricle (*arrow*). **(B)** Coronal T1-weighted image (WI) with contrast shows heterogeneous enhancement of the 4th ventricular mass (*arrow*). **(C)** Sagittal T1WI demonstrates an isointense mass (*arrow*) that occupies the lower aspect of the 4th ventricle. **(D)** Sagittal T1WI with contrast shows the heterogeneous enhancement of the mass (*arrow*).

## Differential Diagnosis

- **Ependymoma:** Sixty percent of intraventricular ependymomas are in the 4th ventricle. They can extend through the foramen of Luschka into the subarachnoid space. They are isodense to brain on noncontrasted computed tomography (CT). Punctate or coarse calcifications are present in 40 to 80%. There is moderate enhancement except for cyst-like regions. Hydrocephalus and hemorrhage are common. There is no gender predilection.
- *Subependymoma:* Subependymomas have no infiltrative pattern. These occur mostly in the 4th ventricle and are usually smaller than 2 cm. Males are more frequently affected. Subependymomas have slight to no enhancement. Thirty percent calcify; coarse calcifications are unusual.
- *Medulloblastoma:* These are hyperdense on CT. They originate in the roof of the 4th ventricle. They have intense enhancement and do not extend through the foramen of Luschka. Calcifications are less common. There is a male predominance. They have early subarachnoid spread.

## Essential Facts

- Sixty percent of ependymomas occur in the posterior fossa.
- They are the third most common tumors of the posterior fossa in children (after pilocytic astrocytomas and medulloblastomas).
- They arise from the floor of the 4th ventricle.
- Supratentorial ependymomas are typically extraventricular, most commonly seen in children. They have a better survival rate.

## Other Imaging Findings

- CT: isodense mass with calcifications
- MRI:
  - T1: isointense
  - T2: slightly hyperintense on pseudocystic areas
  - Hyperintense to cerebrospinal fluid on FLAIR images
  - Mild enhancement

## ✓ Pearls & ✗ Pitfalls

- ✓ If a lesion arises from the floor of the 4th ventricle, favor the diagnosis of ependymoma over medulloblastoma.
- ✓ Ependymomas present in an older age range than do medulloblastomas.
- ✓ Ependymomas are isodense to gray matter on CT, whereas medulloblastomas tend to have a higher attenuation. Most supratentorial ependymomas are extraventricular.

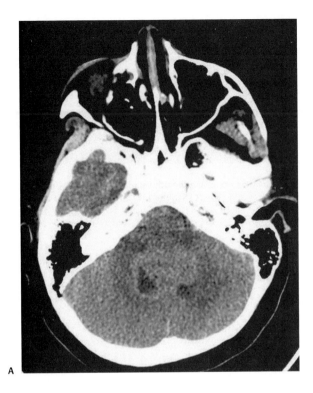

A

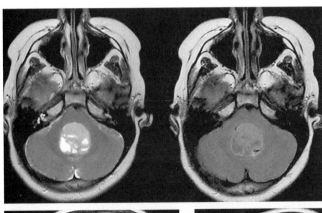

B

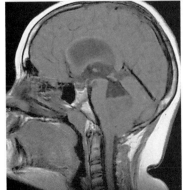

C

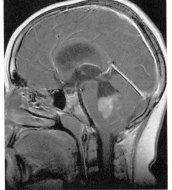

D

# Case 26

## ■ Clinical Presentation

A 7-year-old girl with headaches.

### Further Work-up

## Imaging Findings

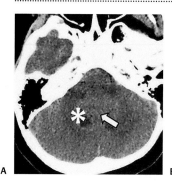 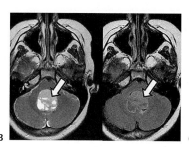 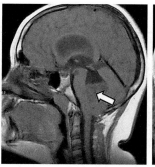 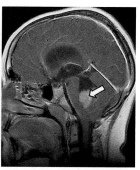

**(A)** Computed tomography (CT) scan of the head without contrast shows a slightly hyperdense mass in the area of the 4th ventricle (*arrow*); there is a cystic part of the lesion (*asterisk*). **(B)** Axial T2-weighted and fluid-attenuated inversion recovery (FLAIR) images show a mass centered in the 4th ventricle that has intermediate signal with cystic components (*arrows*). **(C)** Sagittal T1-weighted image (WI) without contrast shows the mass (*arrow*), which is slightly hypointense to the white matter, occupying the lower aspect of the 4th ventricle. Note the dilatation of the entire ventricular system. **(D)** Sagittal T1WI with contrast shows enhancement of the mass (*arrow*).

## Differential Diagnosis

- **Medulloblastoma:** These are the most common posterior fossa tumors and the second most frequent brain tumors in children (after astrocytomas). They are rare in young adults. Medulloblastomas are highly malignant neuroepithelial tumors. The cerebellum is the most frequent location (95%); most of them occur in the vermis (75%). Hyperattenuation on CT is typical. Medulloblastomas arise from the roof of the 4th ventricle and almost always enhance.
- *Ependymoma:* These are midline cerebellar enhancing masses. Calcifications are frequent (medulloblastomas rarely calcify). They are hypoattenuated on CT (this helps to differentiate them from medulloblastomas). They typically extend through the foramen of Luschka to the subarachnoid space. They arise from the floor of the 4th ventricle (medulloblastomas usually arise from the roof).
- *Pilocytic astrocytoma:* These are the most common pediatric brain tumors. They are cystic with a mural nodule. They have low attenuation on CT (medulloblastomas are typically hyperattenuated). The most common location is the cerebellar hemisphere.

## Essential Facts

- Arise from undifferentiated cells of the posterior medullary velum
- Lateral location more frequent in older children
- Brainstem infiltration in 33%
- Recurrence rates are high.
- World Health Organization grade IV

## Other Imaging Findings

- CT:
  - Well-defined vermian mass
  - Surrounding vasogenic edema (97%)
  - High density because of compact cells (90%)
  - Hydrocephalus
  - Homogeneous enhancement
  - Cyst formation (50%)
  - Rarely calcify (20%)
- Magnetic resonance imaging:
  - Hypointensse relative to white matter on T1-weighted images
  - Heterogeneous on T2WIs
  - High choline peak with reduced *N*-acetylaspartate on spectroscopy

## ✓ Pearls & ✗ Pitfalls

- ✓ Basal nevus syndrome is the association of dural calcifications, keratocysts of the jaw, and medulloblastoma.
- ✓ Some authors suggest that medulloblastomas are infratentorial primitive neuroectodermal tumors, but there is controversy because genetic differences between these tumors have been noted.
- ✗ When a medulloblastoma is diagnosed, scan the entire neuraxis for spinal lesions.
- ✗ Five percent of patients with a medulloblastoma have a concomitant nevoid basal cell carcinoma syndrome.

# Case 27

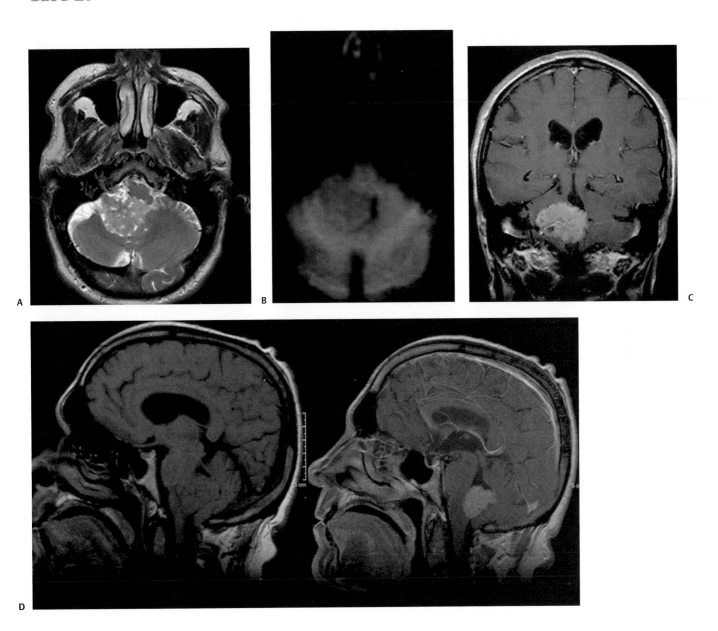

## Clinical Presentation

A 52-year-old with increasing headaches.

## Imaging Findings

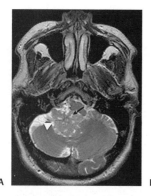
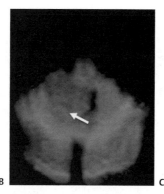
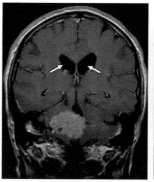
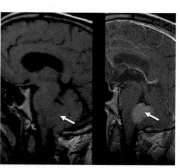

**(A)** Axial T2-weighted image (WI) of the brain shows a heterogeneous mass in the 4th ventricle (*arrow*) that extends to the right cerebellopontine angle (CPA) through the foramen of Luschka (*arrowhead*). **(B)** On axial diffusion-WI, the mass (*arrow*) shows no restriction to diffusion. **(C)** Coronal T1WI with contrast demonstrates avid enhancement of the 4th ventricle mass and dilatation of the lateral ventricles (*arrows*). **(D)** Sagittal T1WIs without and with contrast show a mass with intensity similar to that of the white matter that avidly enhances with gadolinium (*arrows*).

## Differential Diagnosis

- **Choroid plexus papilloma:** These are rare neuroectodermal tumors that account for fewer than 1% of intracranial neoplasms. They are more common in the 4th ventricle in adults, and more common in the atria in children. They are small, cauliflower-like masses with peripheral lobulations. From the 4th ventricle, they may extend through the foramen of Luschka to the subarachnoid space. They have marked enhancement and are associated with hydrocephalus.
- *Medulloblastoma:* These are the most common posterior fossa tumors and the second most frequent brain tumors in children (after astrocytomas). They are rare in young adults. They are highly malignant neuroepithelial tumors. The 4th ventricle is the most frequent location (95%). Hyperattenuation on CT is typical. Medulloblastomas arise from the roof of the 4th ventricle and almost always enhance. They rarely extend to the basal cisterns.
- *Ependymoma:* These are midline cerebellar enhancing masses. Calcifications are frequent. Ependymomas are hypoattenuated on CT. They arise from the floor of the 4th ventricle and typically extend through the foramen of Luschka into the subarachnoid space. They do not have a lobulated appearance.

## Essential Facts

- Choroid plexus papillomas are located where choroid plexus is present.
- The lateral ventricle is the most common site (50%), followed by the 4th ventricle (40%).
- Imaging cannot differentiate choroid plexus papilloma from its histologically aggressive counterpart: choroid plexus carcinoma.

## Other Imaging Findings

- CT:
  - High attenuation with calcifications in 25% of cases
  - Heterogeneous enhancement
- Magnetic resonance imaging:
  - Hypointense on T1 and hyperintense on T2
  - Bright on fluid-attenuated inversion recovery imaging
  - Avid enhancement

## ✓ Pearls & ✗ Pitfalls

- ✓ Seeding can occur with both choroid plexus papillomas and choroid plexus carcinomas.
- ✓ It is necessary to screen the whole neuraxis.
- ✗ The lobulated peripheral appearance is the best way to differentiate choroid plexus papillomas from ependymomas.

# Case 28

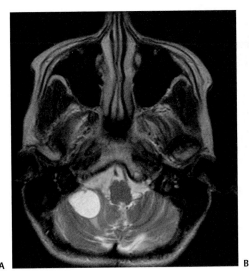
A

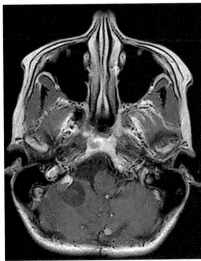
B

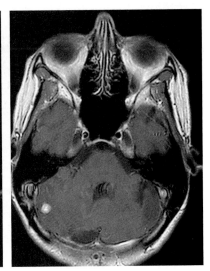
C

## Clinical Presentation

A 54-year-old woman with a recent history of vertigo.

**Further Work-up**

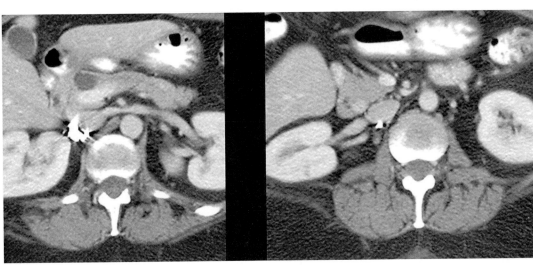
D

### ■ Imaging Findings

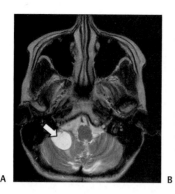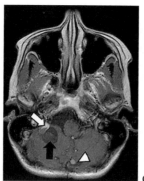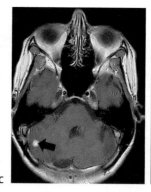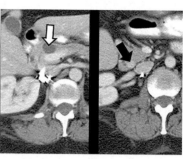

**(A)** Axial T2-weighted image (WI) of the posterior fossa shows a cystic lesion on the right cerebellar hemisphere (*arrow*). There is surrounding vasogenic edema. **(B)** On axial T1WI with contrast, the right cerebellar lesion shows a mural nodule (*white arrow*); the cystic component (*black arrow*) does not enhance. A second enhancing lesion (*arrowhead*) is noted near the midline. **(C)** Axial T1WI of the posterior fossa with contrast shows another enhancing lesion on the left cerebellar hemisphere (*arrow*). **(D)** Axial computed tomography (CT) scans of the abdomen with contrast show a simple pancreatic cyst (*white arrow*). A small enhancing lesion on the pancreatic head is also seen (*black arrow*).

### ■ Differential Diagnosis

- **Cerebellar hemangioblastoma:** These are the most common primary posterior fossa tumors in adults. They appear as an intra-axial cystic mass with a well-defined mural nodule (75%). Of all hemangioblastomas, 4 to 20% are associated with Von Hippel-Lindau (VHL) disease. Eighty percent occur in the cerebellar hemisphere. They displace the 4th ventricle. The mural nodule shows avid enhancement. There are no calcifications.
- *Pilocytic astrocytoma:* These usually occur in children younger than 20 years of age. They appear as a cystic posterior fossa mass with an enhancing nodule. Twenty percent of them calcify. They are located in the cerebellar hemisphere and compress the 4th ventricle.
- *Medulloblastoma:* These are the most common posterior fossa tumors in children. They are highly malignant. They arise from the roof of the 4th ventricle, with an intraventricular location. They appear as a solid mass with cystic degeneration and would rarely present as a cyst with a mural nodule.

### ■ Essential Facts

- Cerebellar hemangioblastomas are rare outside the posterior fossa.
- Up to 40% can be solid tumors.
- The nodule enhances intensely.
- The wall of the cyst rarely enhances.
- The nodule and cyst show high intensity on fluid-attenuated inversion recovery sequences.

### ■ Other Imaging Findings

- CT: the nodule is isodense to brain.

### ✓ Pearls & ✗ Pitfalls

- ✓ Look for other lesions associated with VHL disease, such as other hemangioblastomas, similar lesions in the retina, and renal cell carcinoma.
- ✓ The most frequent posterior fossa mass in adults is metastasis.
- ✓ VHL disease in percentages:
  - Multiple brain hemangioblastomas: 45 to 70%
  - Retinal hemangioblastomas: 50%
  - Renal (70%) and pancreatic (50%) simple cysts
  - Renal cell carcinoma: 30%
  - Pheochromocytoma: 12%
  - Islet cell tumor of the pancreas: 10%

# Case 29

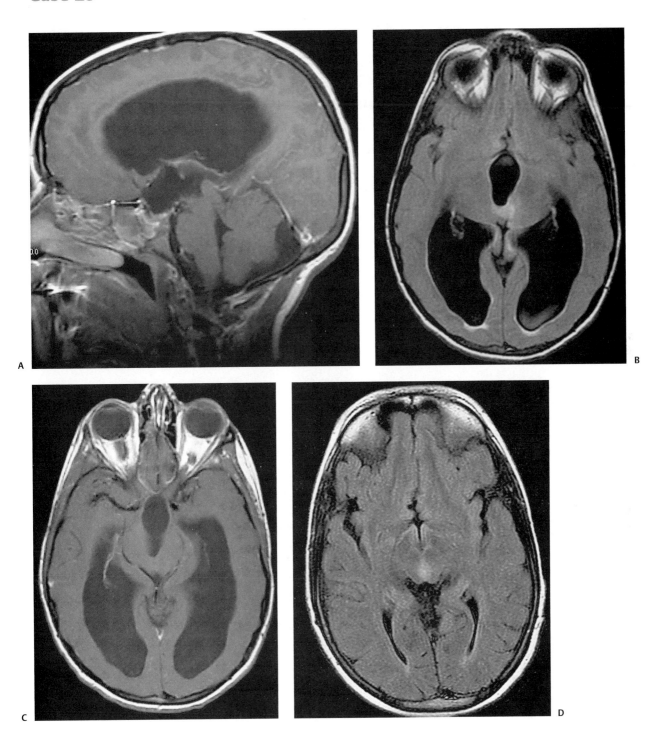

A

B

C

D

## Clinical Presentation

A 12-year-old boy with progressive headaches.

## Imaging Findings

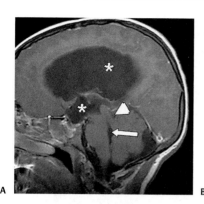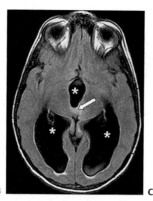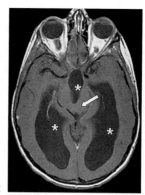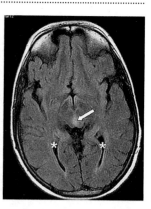

A  B  C  D

**(A)** Sagittal T1-weighted image (WI) shows noncommunicating hydrocephalus with dilated lateral and 3rd ventricles (*asterisks*). The 4th ventricle is not dilated (*arrow*), and the anatomy of the tectum is distorted (*arrowhead*). **(B)** Axial fluid-attenuated inversion recovery (FLAIR) image shows hyperintensity in the midbrain (*arrow*). The lateral and 3rd ventricles are dilated (*asterisks*). **(C)** Axial T1WI with contrast shows no enhancement in the midbrain (*arrow*). Hydrocephalus is seen (*asterisks*). **(D)** Axial FLAIR image shows normal size of the lateral ventricles (*asterisks*) after decompression through a shunt. The area of hyperintensity in the midbrain is again seen (*arrow*).

## Differential Diagnosis

- *Tectal glioma:* These are focal or infiltrative gliomas arising in the tectum. They affect children, usually at 4 to 10 years of age. Early obstruction of the aqueduct can cause hydrocephalus. Calcification is common. Tectal gliomas can grow slowly or show no progression.
- *Hamartoma in neurofibromatosis type 1 (NF1):* The incidence of gliomas and hamartomas is increased in patients with NF1. There is initial growth and enhancement. It is impossible to differentiate hamartoma from tectal glioma by imaging. There is spontaneous regression over time in NF1.
- *Congenital aqueductal stenosis:* This is the most frequent cause of hydrocephalus in the fetus or newborn. Macrocrania is common. There is no mass, FLAIR signal abnormality, or contrast enhancement.

## Essential Facts

- Acquired aqueductal stenosis is the most common manifestation at presentation.
- The pattern of enhancement is variable, but there may be no enhancement.
- Consider a glioma in a young patient with a prominent midbrain and hydrocephalus.

## Other Imaging Findings

- Computed tomography:
  - Calcifications
  - Hydrocephalus
- Magnetic resonance imaging:
  - T1: isointense
  - T2: slightly hyperintense
  - Contrast: variable enhancement
  - FLAIR: best for delineating tumor

## ✓ Pearls & ✗ Pitfalls

- ✓ Tectal gliomas have a better prognosis if associated with NF1.
- ✓ The more pronounced the enhancement at presentation, the worse the prognosis.
- ✗ In patients with NF1, differentiating a tectal glioma from a hamartoma may be difficult.
- ✗ Conservative management, if possible, is urged for these patients.

# Case 30

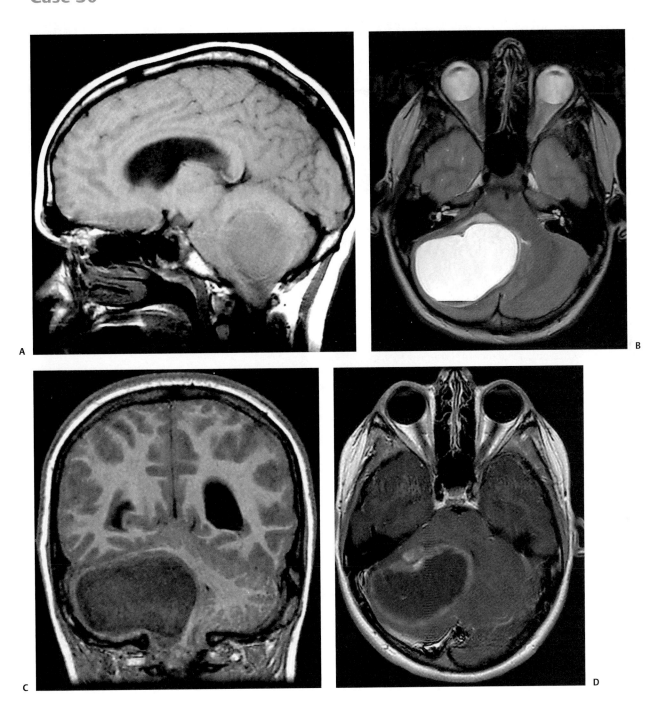

## ■ Clinical Presentation

A 13-year-old boy with a history of gait disturbance and vomiting.

## ■ Imaging Findings

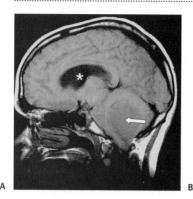 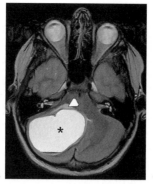 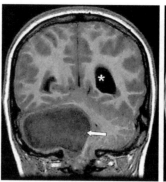 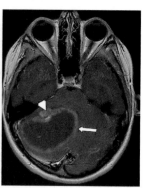

A    B    C    D

**(A)** Sagittal T1-weighted image (WI) shows an enlarged 4th ventricle. A mass (*arrow*) is effacing the 4th ventricle. The lateral ventricles are dilated (*asterisk*). **(B)** Axial T2WI shows a cystic mass centered on the right cerebellar hemisphere (*asterisk*). There is mild surrounding edema (*arrowhead*). **(C)** Coronal T1WI shows the right cerebellar mass (*arrow*) and the dilated lateral ventricle (*asterisk*). **(D)** Axial T1WI with contrast shows peripheral enhancement of the mass (*arrow*); there is an anterior mural nodule (*arrowhead*).

## ■ Differential Diagnosis

- **Pilocytic astrocytoma:** This is the most common pediatric brain tumor (85%). Patients younger than 20 years are affected (75%), with a peak incidence in those 5 to 15 years of age. It appears as a cystic cerebellar mass with a mural nodule. There is low attenuation on computed tomography (CT). The most common location is in the cerebellar hemisphere. It deforms the 4th ventricle.
- *Medulloblastoma:* This is the most common posterior fossa tumor and the second most frequent brain tumor in children (after astrocytoma). It is rare in young adults. It is a highly malignant neuroepithelial tumor. Hyperattenuation on CT is typical. It almost always enhances. Medulloblastoma arises from the roof of the 4th ventricle. Fifty percent have cystic degeneration.
- *Ependymoma:* This is a midline cerebellar enhancing mass. Calcifications are frequent. It is hypoattenuated on CT. It typically extends through the foramen of Luschka into the subarachnoid space. It arises from the floor of the 4th ventricle.

## ■ Essential Facts

- Ten percent of all childhood intracranial neoplasms are pilocytic astrocytomas.
- CT: the cyst is hypodense, the mural nodule is isodense; 20% show calcification.
- Magnetic resonance imaging:
  - T1: low signal
  - T2: high signal of cyst
  - Contrast: enhancement of nodule; possible ring enhancement of cyst
  - Fluid-attenuated inversion recovery: no suppression of cyst

## ✓ Pearls & ✗ Pitfalls

- ✓ Thirty-three percent of patients with a pilocytic astrocytoma involving the optic pathway have neurofibromatosis type 1.
- ✓ Patients with hypothalamic and optic nerve involvement have a worse prognosis.
- ✗ When the optic nerves are involved, the enhancement is variable.
- ✗ A location outside the 4th ventricle can help to differentiate pilocytic astrocytoma from medulloblastoma.
- ✗ Pilocytic astrocytoma is not a likely diagnosis in adults.

# Case 31

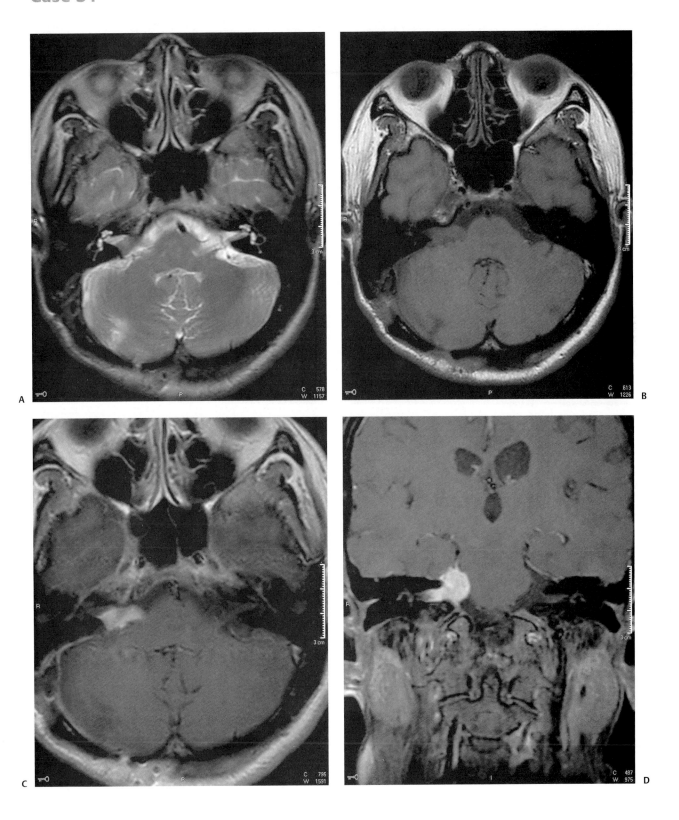

## Clinical Presentation

A 43-year-old man with right-sided progressive hearing loss.

## ■ Imaging Findings

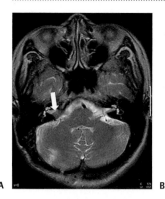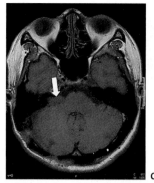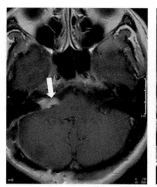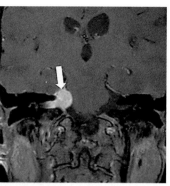

A    B    C    D

**(A)** Axial T2-weighted image (WI) shows expansion of the right internal auditory canal (IAC). A mass is effacing the cerebrospinal fluid (CSF) inside the canal (*arrow*). **(B)** Axial T1WI without contrast shows a mass with intensity similar to that of the brain (*arrow*) in the right IAC and cerebellopontine angle (CPA). **(C)** Axial T1WI with contrast shows intense enhancement of the mass (*arrow*). **(D)** Coronal T1WI with contrast shows the enhancing mass in the right CPA and IAC (*arrow*).

## ■ Differential Diagnosis

- ***Vestibular schwannoma:*** Vestibular schwannomas present as a well-defined mass. They start in the IAC and extend to the CPA. They are the most common CPA mass (85%). They have diffuse enhancement and no dural tail. They expand the IAC, depending on their size. Microhemorrhage can be seen on T2*WIs.
- *Meningioma:* This is a well-defined, avidly enhancing mass with a dural tail. It starts in the CPA and rarely extends through the IAC. Meningiomas account for 10% of CPA tumors (second most common). No microhemorrhage is seen on T2*WIs.
- *Epidermoid cyst:* Epidermoid cysts are the third most common CPA masses. They are ectodermal inclusion cysts composed of epithelial cells that form a keratohyalin matrix as a consequence of desquamation. They engulf vessels and nerves. The cysts follow the CSF on T1 and T2WIs but show signal on fluid-attenuated inversion recovery images. They have a high signal on diffusion-WIs secondary to T2 "shine through." They do not have enhancement.

## ■ Essential Facts

- Consider if there is a unilateral enhancing mass in the CPA in adults.
- There is no extension to the 4th ventricle.
- Magnetic resonance imaging:
  - T1: isointense to brain
  - T2: heavy T2-weighted, high-resolution images good for demonstration
  - T2*: shows microhemorrhage
  - T1 with contrast: avid enhancement
  - Diffusion-WIs: low signal

## ■ Other Imaging Findings

- Computed tomography shows an enlarged ICA (depending on size) with no calcification. The tumor is isodense to brain.

## ✓ Pearls & ✗ Pitfalls

- ✓ The vestibular nerve is more commonly affected than the cochlear nerve, hence the name vestibular schwannoma.
- ✓ Malignant transformation is rare.
- ✓ Vestibular schwannomas are associated with meningiomas in neurofibromatosis type 1.
- ✓ Fifteen percent present with mural cysts.
- ✗ A schwannoma can trap CSF and present with arachnoid cysts.

# Case 32

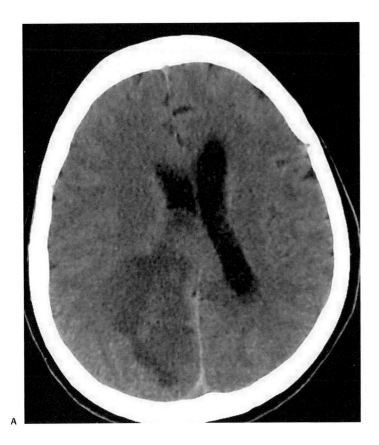

A

## ■ Clinical Presentation

A 64-year-old woman with progressive mental deterioration, nausea, and vomiting.

## Further Work-up

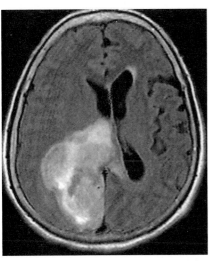

B

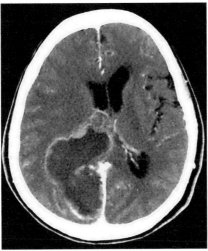

C

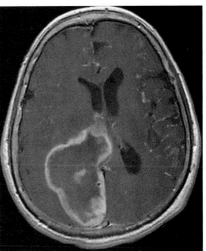

D

### Imaging Findings

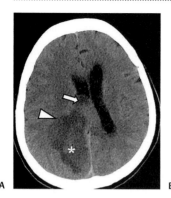 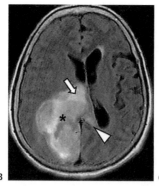 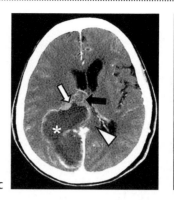 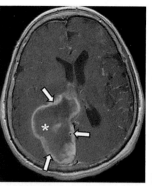

**(A)** Axial computed tomography (CT) scan of the head without contrast shows a low-density mass in the right occipital region (*asterisk*) with an isodense halo (*arrowhead*) and mass effect that effaces the lateral ventricle (*arrow*). **(B)** Axial fluid-attenuated inversion recovery (FLAIR) image shows a heterogeneous mass (*asterisk*) with peripheral high signal that crosses the corpus callosum (*arrowhead*). The mass effaces the lateral ventricle (*arrow*). **(C)** Axial CT scan of the head with contrast shows irregular, thick peripheral enhancement (*white arrow*) and the low-density mass (*asterisk*). The edema crossing the corpus callosum is seen (*arrowhead*). The mass has subependymal extension to the lateral ventricle (*black arrow*). **(D)** Axial T1-weighted image (WI) with contrast shows irregular enhancement (*arrows*) of the right occipital mass (*asterisk*).

### Differential Diagnosis

- *Glioblastoma multiforme (GBM):* GBM is a World Health Organization grade IV astrocytic tumor. It presents as a large, irregular heterogeneous mass with central necrosis and thick peripheral enhancement. It is typically located in the supratentorial white matter, involves the corpus callosum, and causes extensive vasogenic edema. It presents in patients 50 to 70 years old. Calcifications are extremely rare.
- *Solitary metastasis:* These typically are round masses located in the gray-white matter interface, demonstrate vasogenic edema, do not cross commissures, do not restrict diffusion, and are usually multiple.
- *Abscess:* Abscesses are solitary or multiple ring-enhancing lesions with a cystic center. The rim is usually thinner than the rim of GBM. They show restricted diffusion, which helps differentiate them from GBM. They also are associated with vasogenic edema, do not cross commissures, and are located in the gray-white matter interface.

### Essential Facts

- Astrocytomas account for half of primary intracranial neoplasms. Of these, 50% are classified as GBM, making it the *most* common primary intracranial neoplasm.
- The mass effect is extensive.
- If the mass crosses the corpus callosum, it has the typical "butterfly wing" pattern.

### Other Imaging Findings

- CT:
  - Isodense mass with central hypodensity
  - No calcifications
- Magnetic resonance (MR) imaging:
  - T2: heterogeneous mass; necrosis shows high signal
  - FLAIR: high signal of periphery and center of mass; demonstrates vasogenic edema and early extension
  - T1 with contrast: peripheral enhancement, usually thick, can be nodular
  - MR spectroscopy: reversal of Hunter angle with decreased *N*-acetylaspartate and elevated choline peak; increased myoinositol level may be present
  - Diffusion-WIs: no restriction

### ✓ Pearls & ✗ Pitfalls

- ✓ GBM can extend through white matter tracts.
- ✓ Patterns of metastatic spread may be through cerebrospinal fluid, subependymal or hematogenous spread.
- ✓ Tumor goes beyond area of enhancement.
- ✓ Evaluate for mass effect.
- ✗ Associated with genetic syndromes:
  - Turcot syndrome: GBM, colonic adenomatous polyposis, and medulloblastoma
  - Increased incidence in neurofibromatosis type 1
- ✗ Rarely, it can arise in the periphery of the brain, resembling a dura-based process.

# Case 33

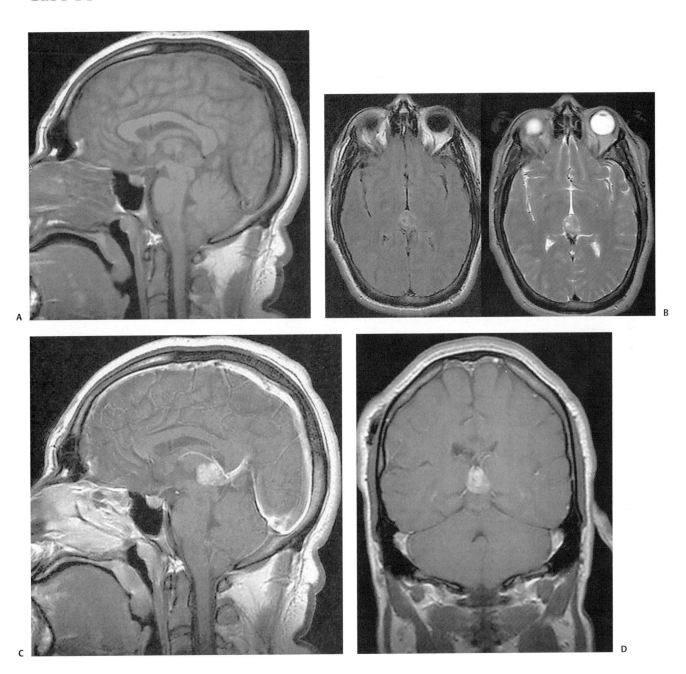

A

B

C

D

## ■ Clinical Presentation

A patient with precocious puberty and limited upward gaze.

### ■ Imaging Findings

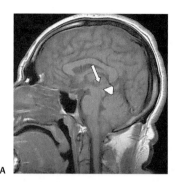 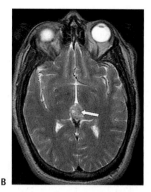 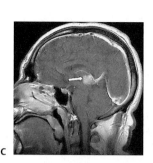 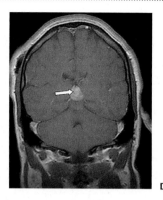

A    B    C    D

**(A)** Sagittal T1-weighted image (WI) shows a mass in the pineal region (*arrow*) compressing the tectum (*arrowhead*). There is a ventricular shunt in place to drain hydrocephalus from aqueductal compression. **(B)** Axial T2WI shows a heterogeneous mass in the pineal region (*arrow*). The mass has punctate areas of hypointensity (calcifications). **(C)** Sagittal T1WI with contrast shows diffuse enhancement of the mass (*arrow*). **(D)** Coronal T1WI with contrast shows the enhancing mass in the pineal region (*arrow*).

### ■ Differential Diagnosis

- **Germinoma:** Germinomas account for two-thirds of pineal region masses. Eighty percent of germinomas occur in the pineal region, and the other 20% occur in the infundibular region. These lesions have a male predominance. They present as hyperdense lesions on computed tomography (CT). Germinomas manifest by the second to third decade of life. Pineal calcification in a child is highly suspicious for germ cell tumor. Germinomas engulf the central calcified gland. They have diffuse enhancement. They are malignant tumors.
- *Pineoblastoma:* These are malignant tumors that are less frequent than germinomas (15% of pineal masses). Pineoblastomas arise from the pineal gland, displacing the calcifications superiorly. There is no gender predilection. Because they have no capsule, they can directly invade the brain or spread to the cerebrospinal fluid (CSF).
- *Teratoma:* These are the second most common tumors of the pineal region. Teratomas are well-circumscribed, multicystic masses that show fat signal. They can have ring enhancement or enhancement limited to the solid component. Calcifications are frequent. There is a male predilection.

### ■ Essential Facts

- Germinomas are not encapsulated masses, which increases the likelihood of drop metastasis.
- Pineal germinomas tend to invade the posterior 3rd ventricle.

### ■ Other Imaging Findings

- Magnetic resonance imaging: iso- or hyperintense to brain on T1, isointense on T2; shows enhancement
- CT: shows calcifications and increased attenuation

### ✓ Pearls & ✗ Pitfalls

- ✓ A CSF study is used to detect increased levels of α-feto-protein, β-human chorionic gonadotropin, and placental alkaline phosphatase; these can indicate the presence of a germ cell tumor.
- ✓ Germ cell tumors include germinomas, teratomas, endodermal sinus tumors, and embryonal carcinomas.
- ✓ Germinoma is the most common pure germ cell tumor.
- ✓ Most of the pineal tumors present with hydrocephalus secondary to compression of the aqueduct.
- ✗ Most solid masses in the pineal region are malignant germ cell tumors.
- ✗ If the mass is multilocular with a lipid signal, favor teratoma (another germ cell tumor).
- ✗ Most of the lesions in the pineal region enhance because there is no blood-brain barrier.

# Case 34

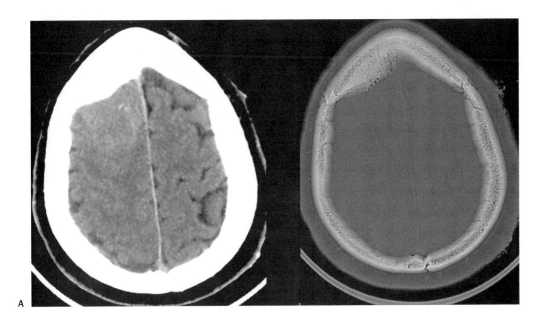

A

## Clinical Presentation

A 48-year-old man with left-sided motor weakness and vomiting.

## Further Work-up

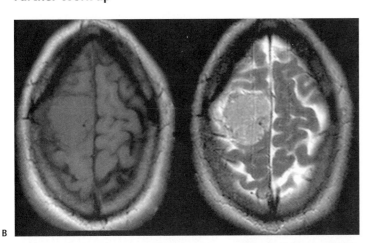

B

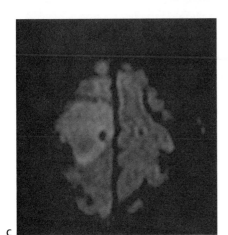

C

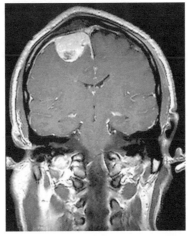

D

### ■ Imaging Findings

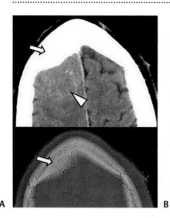
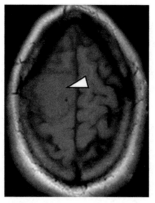
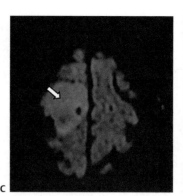
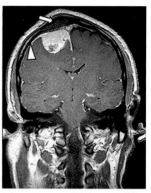

A    B    C    D

**(A)** Axial computed tomography (CT) scan of the head shows a slightly hyperdense lesion in the right frontal region (*arrowhead*) with adjacent cortical thickening (*arrows*). **(B)** Axial T1-weighted image (WI) shows an isointense lesion in the right frontal region (*arrowhead*) that effaces the adjacent sulci. **(C)** Diffusion-WI shows increased signal in the right frontal lesion (*arrow*). **(D)** Coronal T1WI with contrast shows diffuse enhancement of the mass. There is thickening of the adjacent skull (*arrow*). The *arrowhead* shows the dural tail.

### ■ Differential Diagnosis

- ***Meningioma:*** Meningioma is the most common extra-axial intracranial neoplasm. It is a well-circumscribed globular peripheral mass with marked enhancement. It causes "cortical buckling" of the underlying brain and has broad attachment to the dura mater. Calcifications occur in 25% of cases. A dural tail and hyperostosis of the adjacent calvarium are typically seen. Peripheral vasogenic edema occurs in 60% of cases.
- *Epidural metastasis:* This presents as thickening of the dura mater with diffuse enhancement. Extension to the inner table of the skull is common. The lesions are infiltrating rather than well-defined globular lesions with cortical buckling, as in meningioma.

### ■ Essential Facts

- Symptomatic meningiomas are more common in female patients between 40 and 60 years of age.
- Definitions:
  - Typical meningioma: World Health Organization (WHO) grade I
  - Atypical meningioma: WHO grade II
  - Malignant meningioma: WHO grade III

### ■ Other Imaging Findings

- CT: 75% are hyperdense and 25% calcify.
- Magnetic resonance imaging (MRI):
  - T1: isointense to brain
  - T2: variable intensity
  - Fluid-attenuated inversion recovery: best for evaluation of peripheral edema
  - T1 with contrast: diffuse enhancement with dural tail
- Angiogram: Shows the "mother-in-law" sign: "arrives early, leaves late." Evaluate for involvement of venous sinus.

### ✓ Pearls & ✗ Pitfalls

- ✓ Meningiomas can be multiple if associated with mutations.
- ✓ Less frequently, meningiomas may have cystic degeneration, necrosis, or hemorrhage.
- ✗ Always review bone windows on CT to evaluate for cortical thickening, inner table invasion, or fractures.
- ✗ MRI with contrast is the imaging modality of choice for characterizing and evaluating the extent of a meningioma.

# Case 35

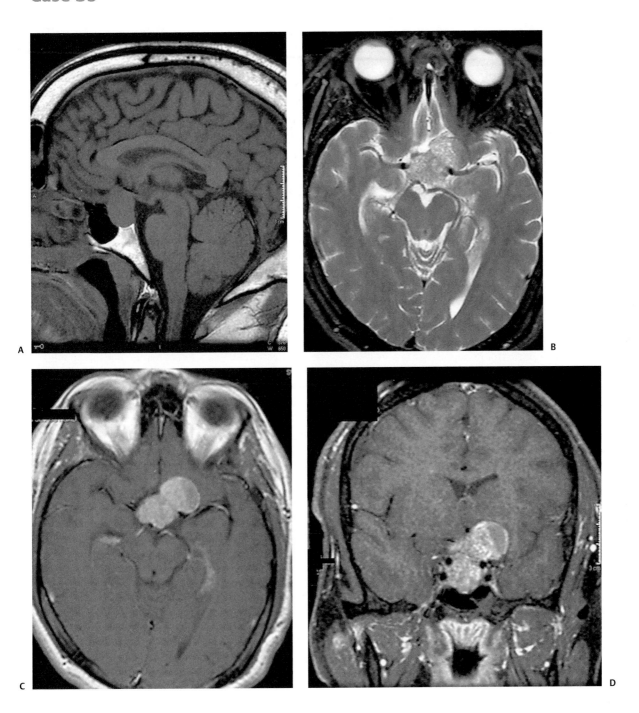

## ■ Clinical Presentation

A 43-year-old with headache and bitemporal hemianopsia.

### ■ Imaging Findings

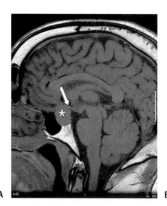 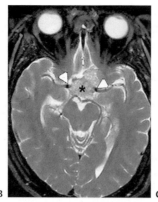 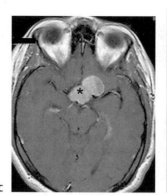 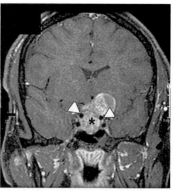

A                      B                      C                      D

**(A)** Sagittal T1-weighted image (WI) shows a sellar mass with suprasellar extension (*asterisk*). The mass is isointense to brain and is displacing the optic chiasm superiorly (*arrow*). **(B)** Axial T2WI shows a heterogeneous mass in the suprasellar region (*asterisk*) that encases the internal carotid arteries without obstructing their flow (*arrowheads*). **(C)** Axial T1WI with contrast shows avid enhancement of the mass (*asterisk*). **(D)** Coronal T1WI with contrast show the encasement of the internal carotid arteries (*arrowheads*) by the mass (*asterisk*).

### ■ Differential Diagnosis

- **Pituitary macroadenoma:** This is a well-defined, enhancing sellar mass that can extend to the suprasellar region. It is a "plastic" tumor that narrows as it crosses the diaphragma sellae, giving the typical "snowman" configuration. Pituitary macroadenomas encase without narrowing the internal carotid arteries. Cavernous extension is common. Central necrosis is seen as cystic formation. There are no calcifications. The mean age at presentation is 20 to 40 years.
- *Craniopharyngioma:* This tumor has a bimodal age distribution, with a first peak in childhood/early adolescence and a second peak in older adults. It is mostly suprasellar; only 21% are intrasellar. Calcifications are typical. Craniopharyngiomas have a cystic component and a solid component that enhances. They have increased signal on precontrast T1WIs.
- *Meningioma:* Sellar region meningiomas start in the suprasellar region and rarely affect the sella. The normal gland can be separated from the lesion. Meningioma enhances avidly and demonstrates a dural tail. Meningioma narrows the internal carotid arteries as it grows. It may calcify.

### ■ Essential Facts

- Pituitary macroadenoma is a benign lesion.
- Ten percent of intracranial neoplasms are pituitary macroadenomas.
- Seventy-five percent have abnormal hormonal activity, usually involving prolactin.
- It is rare in children.
- The capsule of the adenoma represents the normal pituitary gland.

### ■ Other Imaging Findings

- Computed tomography (CT): The sella is widened without calcifications. CT can detect hemorrhage in apoplexy.
- Magnetic resonance imaging:
  - T1: isointense to brain
  - T2: heterogeneous signal, with necrosis appearing as eccentric cyst
  - T1 with contrast: diffuse enhancement
  - Fluid-attenuated inversion recovery: high signal in comparison with brain
  - T2* can detect hemorrhage.

### ✓ Pearls & ✗ Pitfalls

✓ Macroadenomas are said to be "giant" if they exceed 4 cm in diameter.

✓ It is crucial for the clinician to evaluate for cavernous sinus, internal carotid artery, and optic chiasm involvement.

✓ High intensity of the optic nerves has been associated with visual impairment.

✗ It is extremely rare to find a pituitary adenoma that does not involve the sella.

# Case 36

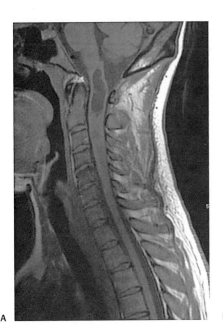

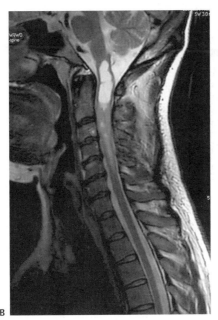

A

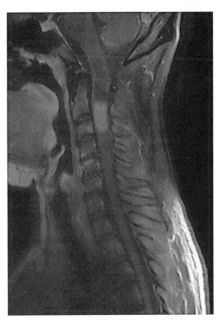

B

C

## Clinical Presentation

A 38-year-old woman with progressive bilateral lower extremity paresthesia.

## Further Work-up

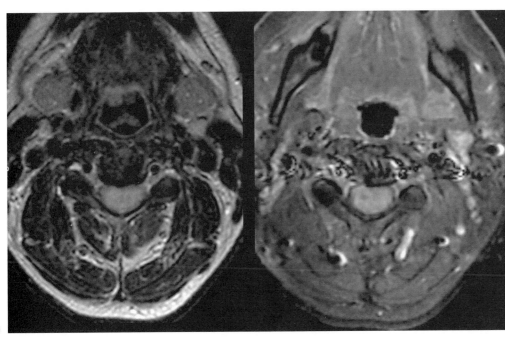

D

### ■ Imaging Findings

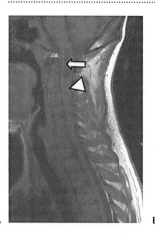
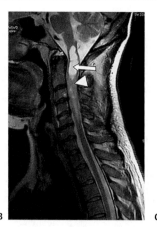
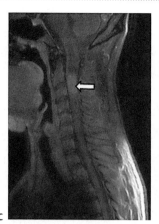
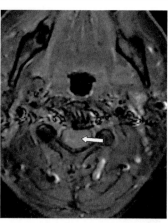

A    B    C    D

**(A)** Axial T1-weighted image (WI) of the cervical spine shows a syrinx (*arrow*) proximal to an ill-defined mass that thickens the spinal cord (*arrowhead*). **(B)** Sagittal T2WI of the cervical spine shows an ill-defined intramedullary mass (*arrowhead*) that is hyperintense to the spinal cord and proximal syringomyelia (*arrow*). **(C)** Sagittal T1WI of the cervical spine with contrast shows an enhancing mass at the C2-C3 level (*arrow*). **(D)** Axial T1WIs of the cervical spine with contrast, without and with fat suppression, show a thickened spinal cord with a diffuse intramedullary enhancing mass (*arrow*).

### ■ Differential Diagnosis

- **Intramedullary astrocytoma:** This accounts for 30% of intraspinal gliomas. It is the most common intramedullary tumor in children and the second most common in adults. The mean age at presentation is 29 years. It is an infiltrating, enhancing tumor, more frequently located in the thoracic cord (70%) and rare in the filum terminale. It tends to be eccentric rather than central and expands the cord. The "cap sign" is not associated with cord astrocytomas.
- *Ependymoma:* This is the most common (60%) of intramedullary tumors in adults. The mean age at presentation is 39 years (10 years later than astrocytomas). Ependymomas are well-defined intraspinal masses, not infiltrative, and more frequently located in the cervical region. They have a central location and are associated with cysts or necrosis. Polar cysts and syrinxes are common. Hemorrhage is common; the "cap sign" is hemosiderin in the cephalic or caudal margin. Spinal canal widening (11%) can occur. They enhance intensely.
- *Hemangioblastoma:* This is an intramedullary enhancing mass. It is associated with Von Hippel-Lindau disease, which is usually located in the posterior aspect of the spinal cord. Hemangioblastomas are adjacent to subpial cysts. Syrinx is less likely because of the eccentric location. They occur most frequently in the thoracic cord. They are typically small lesions. They may have flow voids of prominent vessels.

### ■ Essential Facts

- Patients with intraspinal astrocytomas are less likely to survive than are patients with ependymomas.
- The lesion has poorly defined margins and extends beyond the imaging boundaries.
- Polar and intratumoral cysts and syrinxes are common.
- They span four or fewer spinal segments.

### ■ Other Imaging Findings

- Computed tomography: A thickened spinal cord is associated with syrinx. The spinal canal can be remodeled (less frequent than in ependymomas).
- Magnetic resonance imaging:
  - T1: solid portion isointense to cord, associated cyst/syrinx with low intensity
  - T2: hyperintense
  - T1 with contrast: moderate enhancement with ill-defined borders

### ✓ Pearls & ✗ Pitfalls

- ✓ Can be exophytic
- ✓ Rarely associated with bleeding
- ✗ Fewer than 4% of spinal astrocytomas located in the conus medullaris

# Case 37

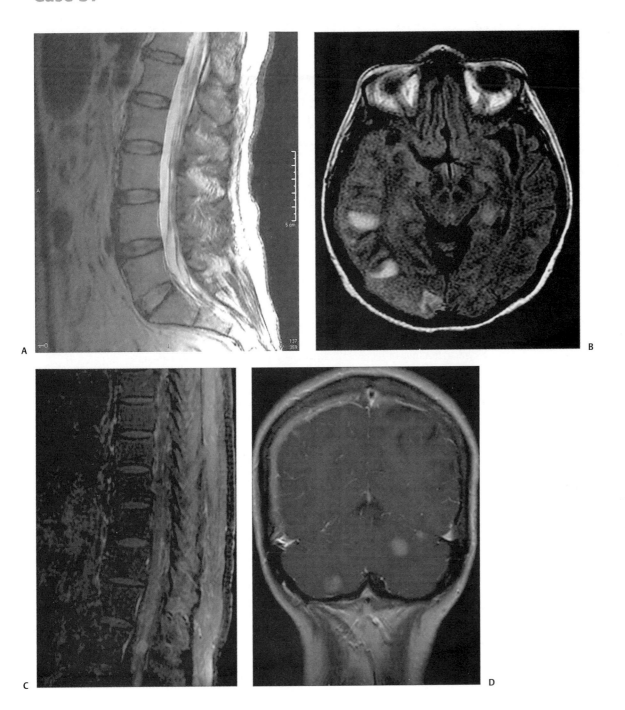

■ **Clinical Presentation**

A 60-year-old woman with the history of a lump in her left breast.

### ◼ Imaging Findings

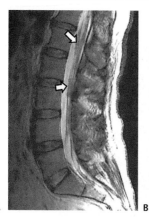
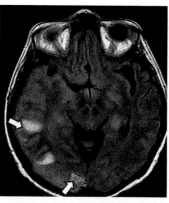
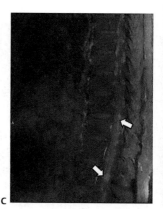
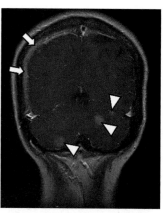

**(A)** Sagittal T2-weighted image (WI) of the lumbar spine shows nodular thickening of the nerve roots (*arrows*). **(B)** Axial fluid-attenuated inversion recovery (FLAIR) image of the brain shows three foci of increased signal in the subcortical white matter on the right (*arrows*). **(C)** Sagittal T1WI of the spine after contrast with fat saturation shows diffuse nodular enhancement of the nerve roots (*arrows*). **(D)** Coronal T1WI of the brain with contrast shows thick meningeal enhancement on the right (*arrows*) along with foci of nodular enhancement in the posterior fossa (*arrowheads*).

### ◼ Differential Diagnosis

- **Meningeal carcinomatosis:** "Sugarcoating" and nodular enhancement of the nerve roots are typical findings of meningeal carcinomatosis. It can result from hematogenous spread of extracranial disease or from "drop" metastasis of intracranial disease. It often causes thickening of the nerve roots. The conus medullaris is also involved. The entire neuraxis should be assessed.
- *Meningitis and cerebritis:* The combination of leptomeningeal enhancement and brain parenchymal lesions can be the result of infection, leading to this diagnosis.

### ◼ Essential Facts

- Meningeal carcinomatosis can be secondary to metastasis from primary tumors of the central nervous system or from distant tumors.
- Cytology of the cerebrospinal fluid is useful to confirm the diagnosis.
- Hematogenous brain metastases are typically located in the subcortical white matter.
- Tumors that typically have leptomeningeal spread include lung carcinoma, breast carcinoma, and lymphoma.
- Meningeal metastases tend to be isointense to gray matter, so that they are hard to identify without contrast.
- Nodular enhancement of the nerve roots is typical.
- FLAIR can show increased signal in the sulci of patients with meningeal carcinomatosis; however, this does not help to differentiate it from meningitis.

### ✓ Pearls & ✘ Pitfalls

- ✓ Remember to scan the entire neuraxis in patients with suspected meningeal carcinomatosis.
- ✓ Skull involvement is possible and appears as an enhancing lesion invading the diploic space.
- ✓ Diffusion-WIs will be bright in hematogenous parenchymal abscesses and can help differentiate them from metastases.
- ✘ Both magnetic resonance imaging with contrast and cerebrospinal fluid analysis yield false-negative results for the detection of leptomeningeal carcinomatosis and should be used in combination to increase their sensitivity.

# Case 38

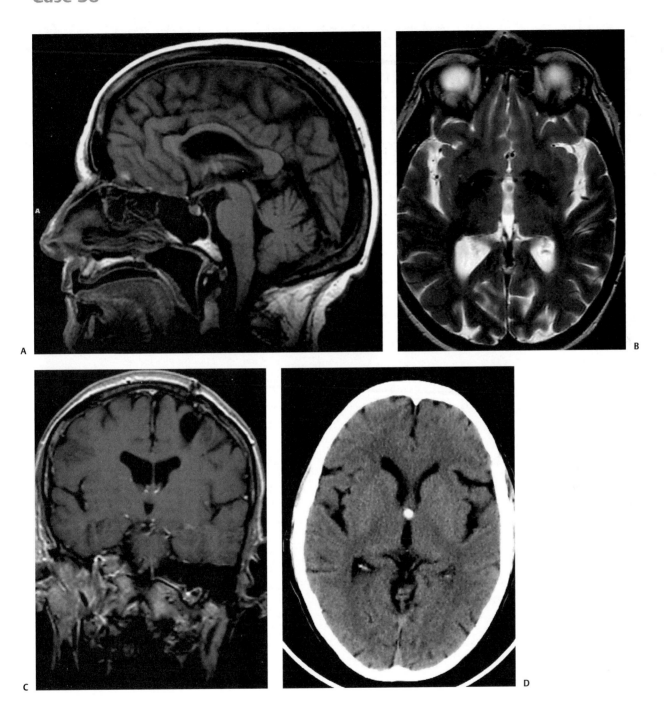

## Clinical Presentation

An adult woman with severe intermittent headaches.

## Imaging Findings

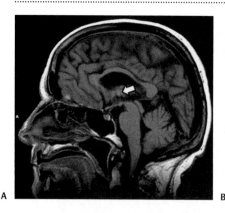 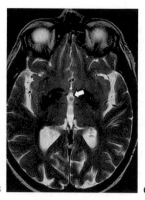 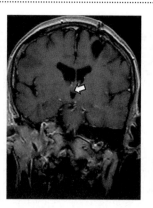 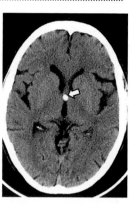

**(A)** Sagittal T1-weighted image (WI) shows a round mass in the roof of the 3rd ventricle (*arrow*). The mass is isointense to the gray matter. **(B)** Axial T2WI shows the lesion as isointense to cerebrospinal fluid (*arrow*). **(C)** Coronal T1WI with contrast shows the lesion in the roof of the 3rd ventricle (*arrow*); there is no enhancement. **(D)** Computed tomography (CT) of the head without contrast shows a hyperdense lesion in the 3rd ventricle (*arrow*) adjacent to the anterior pillars of the fornix.

## Differential Diagnosis

- **Colloidal cyst:** Colloidal cysts are histologically benign lesions attached to the roof of the 3rd ventricle. They obstruct the foramen of Monro and cause hydrocephalus. They do not have enhancement or calcifications.
- *Flow artifact:* Flow artifact in the foramen of Monro on fluid-attenuated inversion recovery and T2WIs is usually seen in the lateral ventricles, not the 3rd ventricle. This is not seen on CT or magnetic resonance (MR) sequences with a short echo time. There is no hydrocephalus.

## Essential Facts

- Benign cysts are characterized histologically by an epithelial lining with mucous goblet cells.
- They apparently originate from the endoderm, sharing characteristics with Rathke cleft cysts.
- Most colloidal cysts are hyperdense on CT.
- The MR appearance is variable, and the cysts can be difficult to identify.
- Half of them show increased T1 signal.
- There is no enhancement.

## ✓ Pearls & ✗ Pitfalls

- ✓ Many small colloidal cysts can be hard to identify on MR. CT without contrast can be the best diagnostic modality in these cases.
- ✗ Rarely, colloid cysts can present with rim enhancement.

# Case 39

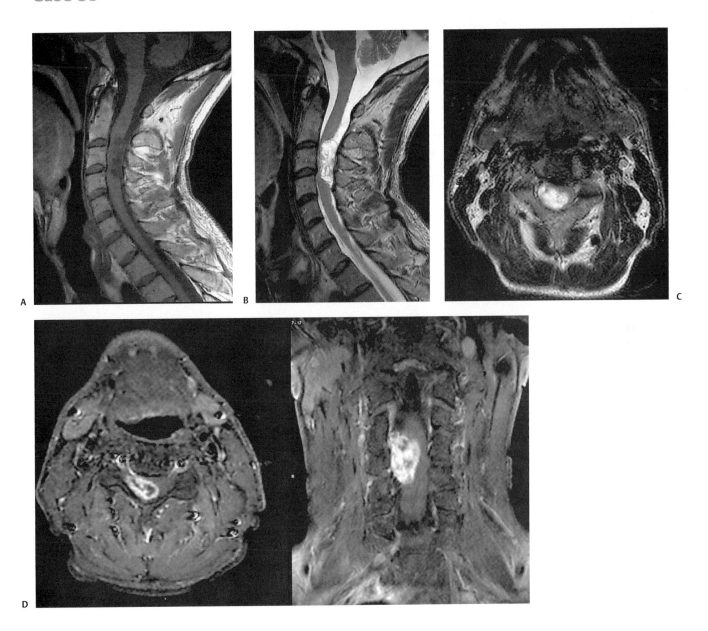

A

B

C

D

## Clinical Presentation

A 27-year-old woman with progressive paresthesia in the right shoulder and arm.

■ **Imaging Findings**

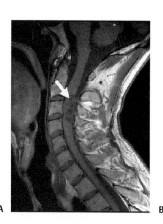
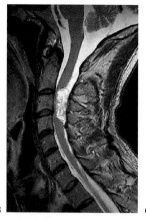
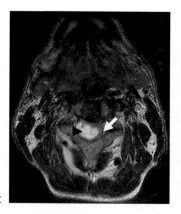
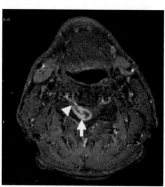

**(A)** Sagittal T1-weighted image (WI) of the cervical spine shows a low-signal lesion at the level of C3 (*arrow*). The lesion is extra-axial. **(B)** Sagittal T2WI of the cervical spine shows high signal of the mass. **(C)** Axial T2WI shows the mass (*arrowhead*) in the right aspect of the intradural space. The lesion compresses the spinal cord (*arrow*). **(D)** Axial fat-saturated T1WI of the cervical spine with contrast shows the "target" pattern of enhancement of the intradural, extramedullary mass (*arrow*). The lesion extends to the right neural foramen (*arrowhead*).

■ **Differential Diagnosis**

- **Spinal schwannoma:** Spinal schwannomas comprise 80% of intradural extramedullary masses. They usually have an anterior and lateral location in the spinal canal. They extend to the neural foramen and enlarge it. They often compress the spinal cord. These lesions are typically solitary (unless they are related to neurofibromatosis type 2), demonstrate avid enhancement (which can have a "target" appearance), and do not calcify.
- *Meningioma:* Meningiomas are the second most common intradural extramedullary masses. They are localized in the posterior and lateral aspect of the spinal canal, more frequently at the thoracic level. They show intense enhancement and do not extend to the neural foramen. They may have a dural tail. Calcifications are rare.
- *Neurofibroma:* This presents as multiple masses exiting the neural foramina as part of neurofibromatosis type 1. Neurofibromas affect multiple levels, enhance intensely, and expand the neural foramina. When a lesion is solitary, it is impossible to differentiate it from a schwannoma.

■ **Essential Facts**

- Schwannoma is the most common intradural extramedullary mass.
- Schwannoma can have fatty degeneration, cystic degeneration, or hemorrhage.
- Intensity is low on T1WIs and high on T2WIs in comparison with the spinal cord. There is a characteristic change if fatty or cystic degeneration is present.
- Enhancement is intense; the "target sign" (low central signal along with peripheral enhancement) may be seen.

■ **Other Imaging Findings**

- Schwannomas are isodense to the spinal cord on computed tomography.

✓ **Pearls & ✗ Pitfalls**

- ✓ Schwannoma is the most common intradural extramedullary mass.
- ✓ The location is important: schwannomas tend to be anterior and lateral, whereas meningiomas are posterior.
- ✗ No bony erosions are seen with schwannomas.

# Case 40

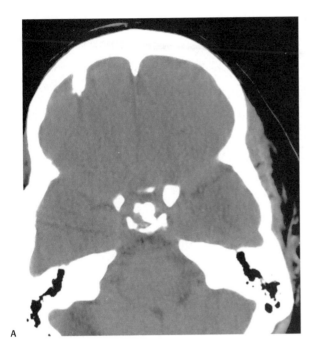

A

## Clinical Presentation

A 40-year-old woman with severe headache and blurry vision.

## Further Work-up

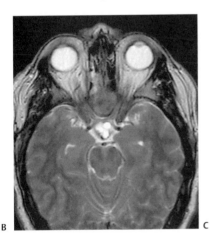

B

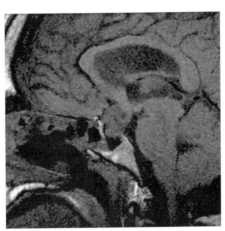

C

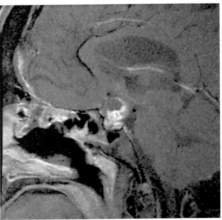

D

### ■ Imaging Findings

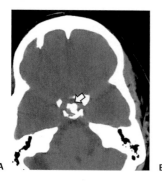 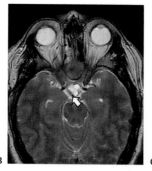 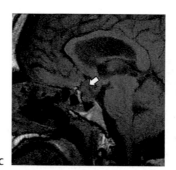 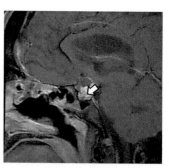

A          B          C          D

**(A)** Axial computed tomography scan of the brain shows irregular calcifications in the supraclinoid region (*arrow*). **(B)** On axial T2-weighted image (WI), the lesion has a multiloculated appearance. Note the dark posterior rim arising from calcification (*arrow*). **(C)** Sagittal T1WI shows sellar and suprasellar components of the mass, which is heterogeneous in signal (*arrow*). **(D)** Sagittal T1WI after gadolinium injection shows enhancement in the solid areas of the tumor (*arrow*) and nonenhancing cystic areas.

### ■ Differential Diagnosis

- **Craniopharyngioma:** This is a suprasellar mass with a mixed solid and cystic appearance. It shows reticulated enhancement after the administration of gadolinium. It has a mass effect on the floor of the 3rd ventricle and hypothalamus.
- *Rathke cleft cyst:* This is a benign epithelium-lined cyst that is thought to be a remnant of the Rathke pouch. Seventy percent of Rathke cleft cysts involve both intrasellar and suprasellar regions. It is a cystic lesion, with a smooth margin and homogeneous signal intensity. It may have a high T1 signal with a thin rim or no enhancement.
- *Pituitary adenoma:* This is the most common of the lesions involving both the intrasellar and suprasellar regions. Pituitary adenomas arise from the pituitary gland and extend through the diaphragma sellae up toward the optic chiasm. They are isointense to gray matter and show homogeneously intense enhancement after gadolinium administration. Necrosis, cystic degeneration, and hemorrhage are not uncommon. Pituitary adenomas with suprasellar extension typically have a "figure of eight" or "snowman" appearance.

### ■ Essential Facts

- Craniopharyngiomas are epithelial neoplasms arising from squamous epithelial rests of the Rathke pouch.
- The clinical presentation includes visual disturbance, endocrine dysfunction, and raised intracranial pressure.
- The distribution by age is bimodal, with a peak incidence in children 5 to 14 years of age and again in adults 65 to 74 years of age.

### ■ Other Imaging Findings

- Magnetic resonance (MR) imaging:
  - Suprasellar (75%), suprasellar and infrasellar (20%), and infrasellar (5%) regions
  - Partly solid, partly cystic, calcified mass lesion
  - Reticular enhancement in the solid portion
  - Superior extension compressing the 3rd ventricle
- MR angiography is useful to delineate the course of the vessels.

### ✓ Pearls & ✗ Pitfalls

- ✓ Lateral extension beyond the lateral wall of the internal carotid artery may be seen in adenomas and craniopharyngiomas, but not in Rathke cleft cysts.
- ✗ High T1 signal within the cystic component of a craniopharyngioma, adenoma, or Rathke cleft cyst may mimic pituitary apoplexy.

# Case 41

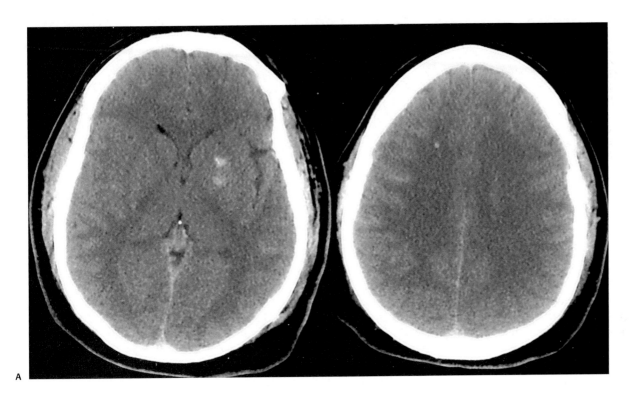

A

## Clinical Presentation

A young woman presenting with loss of consciousness after being involved in a motor vehicle collision.

## Further Work-up

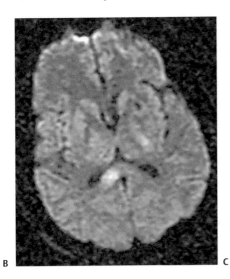

B

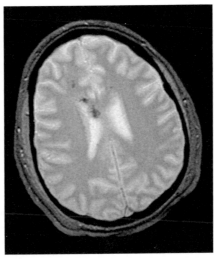

C

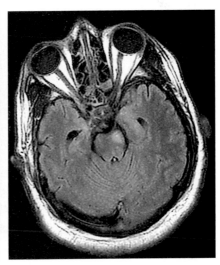

D

## ■ Imaging Findings

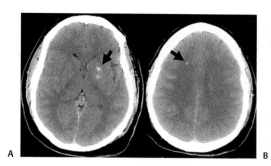
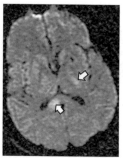
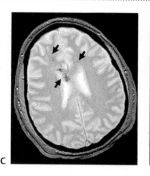
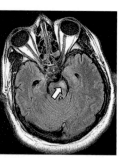

**(A)** Computed tomography (CT) scan of the brain demonstrates multiple punctate foci of hemorrhage in the left basal ganglia and right frontal deep white matter (*arrows*). **(B)** Diffusion-weighted image (WI) shows restricted diffusion in the left basal ganglia and in the splenium of the corpus callosum (*arrows*). **(C)** Petechial hemorrhage in the deep white matter and corpus callosum is evident in the gradient-echo (GRE) T2*WI (*arrows*). Multiple other foci were demonstrated in the brainstem and centrum semiovale. **(D)** Fluid-attenuated inversion recovery image shows increased signal in the left cerebral peduncle (*arrow*).

## ■ Differential Diagnosis

- **Diffuse axonal injury (DAI):** This presents with significant impairment of mental status and relatively scarce CT abnormalities. It is characterized by multiple small hemorrhages in the deep white matter, including the corpus callosum and brainstem.
- *Cerebral contusions:* These are more frequent in the frontal and temporal lobes and are usually adjacent to the skull. Edema may precede hemorrhage by a few hours.
- *Cerebral amyloid angiopathy:* This presents as spontaneous cortical-subcortical intracranial hemorrhage in the normotensive elderly. The intracranial hemorrhage generally spares the deep white matter, basal ganglia, and brainstem. It may involve the cerebellum. Microhemorrhages are visualized on T2*-weighted GRE magnetic resonance (MR) imaging.

## ■ Essential Facts

- DAI is a frequent cause of morbidity in patients with traumatic brain injuries, most commonly injuries resulting from high-speed motor vehicle accidents.
- The traumatic deceleration impact produces rotational forces that injure the areas where the density difference is greatest.
- Two-thirds of DAI lesions occur at the gray-white matter junction. The corpus callosum, dorsolateral rostral brainstem, caudate nucleus, thalamus, tegmentum, and internal capsule are also affected.

## ■ Other Imaging Findings

- CT:
  - Normal CT scan at presentation in 50 to 80% of patients
  - One or more areas of hemorrhage smaller than 2 cm in diameter in the cerebral hemispheres or adjacent to the 3rd ventricle
  - Intraventricular hemorrhage
  - Hemorrhage in the corpus callosum
  - Brainstem hemorrhage
- MR imaging:
  - Diffusion-WIs: hyperintensity in areas of axonal injury
  - GRE T2*WIs: petechial hemorrhages; can persist for many years after the injury
  - T2WIs: multifocal areas of high signal at the white matter in the temporal or parietal corticomedullary junction, corpus callosum, dorsolateral rostral midbrain, and corona radiata
- MR spectroscopy may show diffusely elevated lactate levels, even in tissues that appear normal on MR imaging; these correlate with a poor clinical outcome.

## ✓ Pearls & ✗ Pitfalls

- ✓ It is now recommended that all patients with moderate to severe head injury undergo an MRI examination within the first 2 weeks after the injury for a better evaluation of the full extent of brain involvement, which is not feasible by CT alone.
- ✗ The CT assessment of the brainstem and posterior fossa is limited because of beam-hardening artifacts from bone.
- ✗ Artifacts from the frontal or temporal bones in the GRE T2* sequence limit the assessment of microhemorrhages in these regions.

# Case 42

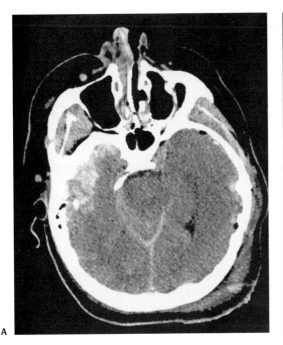
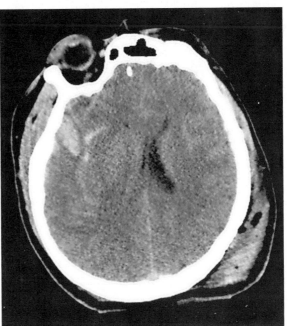

A      B

## ■ Clinical Presentation

A 35-year-old who fell from a height of 14 feet.

## Further Work-up

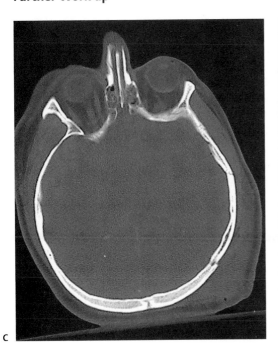
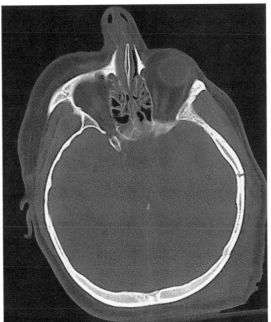

C      D

### ◼ Imaging Findings

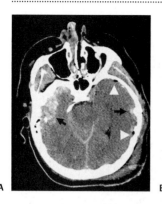
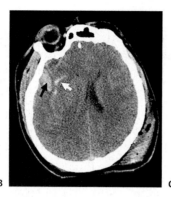
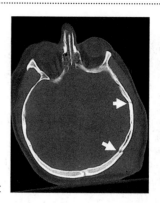
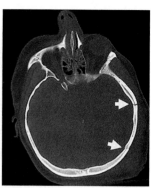

**(A)** Computed tomography (CT) of the brain shows contusions (*arrows*) and subarachnoid hemorrhage in both temporal lobes, which are more extensive on the left. Pneumocephalus (*arrowheads*) and soft-tissue swelling are present only on the left side. **(B)** CT of the brain shows contusion (*black arrow*) and subarachnoid hemorrhage (*white arrow*) in the right temporal lobe. Note the soft-tissue injuries on the left side. **(C,D)** Bone windows display fractures in the left temporal bone (*arrows*).

### ◼ Differential Diagnosis

- ***Coup and contrecoup cerebral injuries:*** These injuries show parenchymal contusions and extra-axial hemorrhages adjacent to the site of injury and in the opposite side of the brain. The contralateral parenchymal injuries tend to be more severe.
- *Bilateral direct trauma:* This is feasible in motor vehicle accidents. It presents with bilateral soft-tissue injuries.
- *Aneurysmal rupture with subsequent fall:* The traumatic lesions are disproportionate for this mechanism of injury. The aneurysmal subarachnoid hemorrhage is usually around the circle of Willis.

### ◼ Essential Facts

- Coup and contrecoup cerebral injuries are acceleration or deceleration injuries of the brain.
- The coup injury occurs at the site of the primary impact, which is identified by the associated scalp injuries or skull fractures.
- Epidural hematoma, contusion, or laceration of the brain surface often occurs at the site of a fracture, especially if it is depressed.
- The contrecoup injury arises on the side opposite the coup injury. Hemorrhagic cerebral contusions are more common and tend be larger on the side of the contrecoup injury, although both coup and contrecoup injuries can be hemorrhagic.

- A severe impact on a stationary head (e.g., a blow with a blunt object) results in skull fractures but generally does not cause contrecoup contusions. This is because, in such cases, the head does not accelerate or decelerate, and there is no brain lag.
- With frontal impact trauma, the brain moves over the floor of the anterior cranial fossa and slams into the sphenoid wings and petrous ridges, with resultant contusions in the inferior frontal, anterior temporal, and lateral temporal regions. Paramedian bony irregularities may cause superior frontal and parasagittal contusions.

### ✓ Pearls & ✗ Pitfalls

- ✓ Repeated imaging is indicated to monitor the size of the hemorrhage and the development of delayed hemorrhage and vasogenic edema.
- ✓ Large hemorrhagic contusions commonly increase in size within the first 48 hours.
- ✗ Contusions in the floor of the anterior cranial fossa and above the petrous ridge can be masked by volume averaging of the adjacent bone. In follow-up images, as edema develops, these contusions become evident.

# Case 43

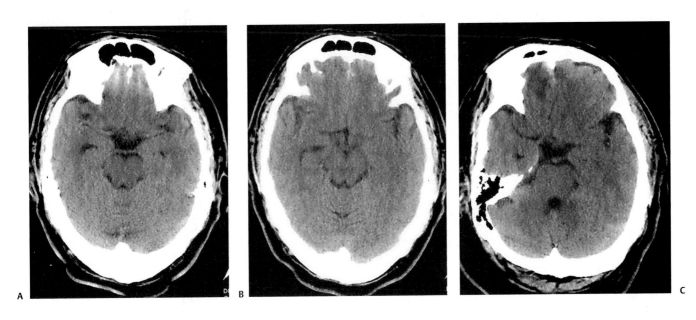

■ **Clinical Presentation**

A 35-year-old with headaches following an assault.

## ■ Imaging Findings

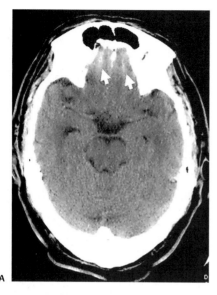
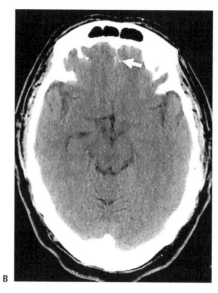
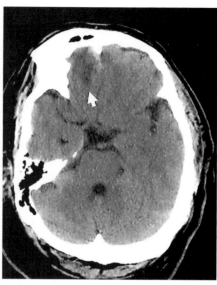

**(A)** Computed tomography (CT) demonstrates increased attenuation along the inferior frontal sulci (*arrows*). No fracture was identified in the images with bone algorithm. **(B)** CT demonstrates increased attenuation in the interhemispheric region (*arrow*). **(C)** Follow-up CT 2 days later shows low attenuation in the right frontal lobe inferiorly, consistent with edema (*white arrow*). The hemorrhage is still visible.

## ■ Differential Diagnosis

- **Traumatic subarachnoid hemorrhage (SAH):** On CT, this shows high-attenuation blood within the basal cisterns and subarachnoid spaces. Traumatic hemorrhage is located in the convexities more frequently than in the basal cisterns. Nonvisualization of the interpeduncular cistern may be a clue that a small amount of isodense subarachnoid blood is present.
- *Aneurysmal SAH:* This presents as severe headache, described as the "worst headache of one's life." Hemorrhage tends to be located near the ruptured aneurysm, around the circle of Willis.
- *Hemorrhagic contusion of the frontal lobe:* This may be difficult to differentiate from and may coexist with SAH. It can be masked by volume averaging with the bone in the floor of the anterior cranial fossa.

## ■ Essential Facts

- Small, bridging cortical vessels on the pia or arachnoidal leptomeninges crossing the subarachnoid space are injured.
- Blood from an intracerebral hematoma may decompress directly into the subarachnoid space or dissect into the ventricular system.
- When SAH occurs in conjunction with other forms of traumatic brain injury, it is often focal and located next to a contusion.
- The most frequent location is the convexity, followed by the fissures and basal cisterns.

- Hydrocephalus is the most common complication after SAH.
- SAH may induce cerebral vasospasm, which is more likely to occur when SAH is accompanied by subdural hematoma, intraventricular hemorrhage, cerebral contusion, or intracerebral hemorrhage.

## ■ Other Imaging Findings

- Fluid-attenuated inversion recovery imaging (FLAIR) images may detect small areas of acute or subacute SAH that are not detected by other magnetic resonance imaging sequences or CT scans.

## ✓ Pearls & ✗ Pitfalls

- ✓ The FLAIR sequence suppresses the intensity of cerebrospinal fluid (CSF) but does not differentiate between abnormalities that appear as high signal intensity: hemorrhage, inflammatory exudate, neoplastic leptomeningeal infiltration, vascular slow flow, and hyperoxygenation during sedation or anesthesia.
- ✗ In the setting of diffuse brain swelling, the elevated intracranial pressure causes an increase in the density of the subarachnoid space (pseudo-SAH) on CT by two mechanisms:
  - The subarachnoid space contracts, and the amount of CSF in that space is decreased.
  - The small pial vessels in the subarachnoid space become engorged and dilated, and a resultant increase in the blood pool contributes to the CT density.

# Case 44

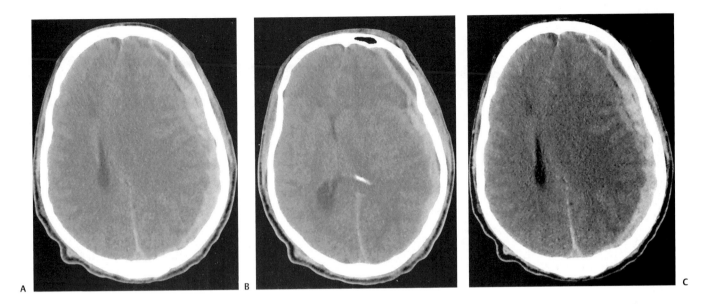

## Clinical Presentation

A 51-year-old man after a motor vehicle collision.

## ▦ Imaging Findings

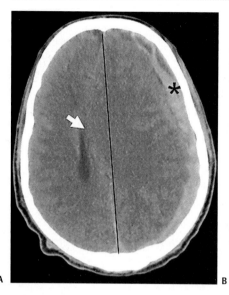
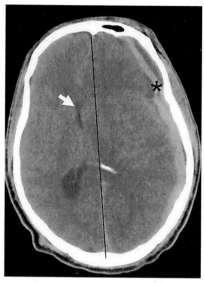
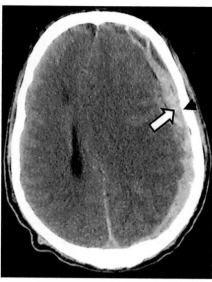

A  B  C

**(A,B)** Computed tomography (CT) scans with "brain windows" reveal a crescent-shaped extra-axial collection with high attenuation that is slightly heterogeneous (*asterisk*). It compresses the left lateral ventricle and causes rightward deviation of the midline structures (*arrow*). **(C)** Note the increased contrast between the hematoma (*arrow*) and the skull (*arrowhead*) in the "blood" window.

## ▦ Differential Diagnosis

- *Acute subdural hematoma (SDH):* Acute SDH is a crescentic, hyperdense collection between the dura and arachnoid membrane. Displacement of the cortex away from the inner table is common. It can cause midline shift with compression of the ipsilateral lateral ventricle and dilatation of the contralateral ventricle.
- *Epidural hematoma:* This is a collection of blood between the inner skull table and the dura. There is an adjacent skull fracture in 90% of cases. On CT, there is a hyperattenuating collection with a biconvex or lenticular shape and sharp margination. A low-attenuation swirl may be the result of blood from active bleeding mixing with serum from clotted blood.
- *Subdural hygroma:* This is a cerebrospinal fluid (CSF) collection that develops 6 to 30 days after a traumatic arachnoid tear. On CT, subdural hygromas have the same density as CSF. Blood vessels crossing through the extra-axial collection help differentiate subdural hygromas from chronic SDHs.

## ▦ Essential Facts

- SDH is a collection of blood between the dura and arachnoid membrane.
- Bleeding may be from cerebral veins, venous sinuses, or cerebral contusions.
- Cerebral contusions are frequently associated with SDHs.
- The mass effect of the collection is greater than expected because of swelling of the hemisphere.
- The most common locations are along the cerebral convexities, the falx cerebri, and the tentorium cerebelli.

- Bilateral SDHs may have a balancing effect, so that there is no midline shift despite significant mass effect.
- Small SDHs may be missed because of high convexity locations, beam-hardening artifacts, or narrow window settings.
- A wider "blood" window (width, 200; level, 70) helps to differentiate pixels of similar brightness and so differentiate acute blood from bone.

## ▦ Other Imaging Findings

- Magnetic resonance imaging (MRI) is more sensitive than CT in the detection of small SDHs and tentorial or interhemispheric SDHs.
- The detection of SDH is critical in cases of suspected child abuse.

## ✓ Pearls & ✗ Pitfalls

- ✓ SDHs may cross suture lines but not dural reflections, such as the falx and tentorium.
- ✓ SDHs that are only a few hours old can have a mixed appearance of both hyperdense and hypodense regions because of the presence of uncoagulated blood before clot formation.
- ✗ In the setting of severe anemia, acute SDHs can be isodense to gray matter.
- ✗ An ossified cerebral falx contains bone marrow with a high T1 signal, which may mimic a subdural hematoma on MRI.

# Case 45

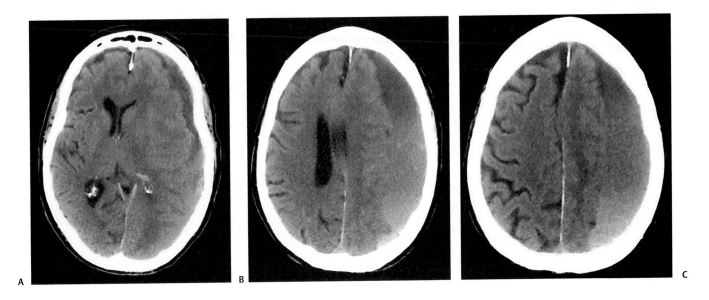

A       B       C

## ▇ Clinical Presentation

A 65-year-old with headache and slow, progressive intellectual decline.

### ■ Imaging Findings

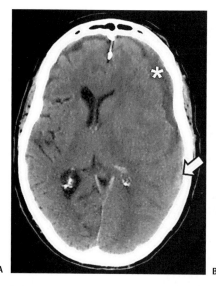
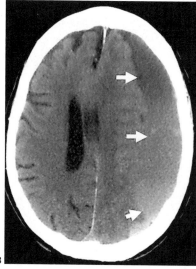
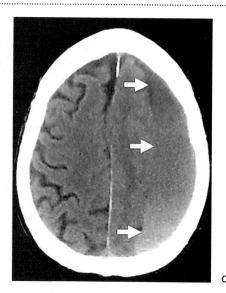

**(A)** Computed tomography (CT) at the level of the lateral ventricles shows a crescent-shaped extra-axial collection in the left convexity with high attenuation in the dependent portion (*arrow*) and fluid attenuation anteriorly (*asterisk*). **(B,C)** The slices in the superior aspect of the brain show a large collection (*arrows*) with layering of blood products causing hematocrit effect. Note the relatively minimal mass effect for the size of the hematoma.

### ■ Differential Diagnosis

- ***Acute-on-chronic subdural hematoma (SDH):*** This is characterized by repeated hemorrhage into previous subdural collections. It may show layering of blood products.
- *Acute SDH:* The mass effect from a collection that develops acutely is much more severe than that of a slowly accumulating hematoma.
- *Epidural hematoma with active bleeding:* This is a biconvex, hyperdense extra-axial fluid collection. There is adjacent skull fracture in 90% of cases. Epidural hematoma with active hemorrhage may contain alternating crescent-shaped regions of various densities that produce a "swirled" appearance.

### ■ Essential Facts

- Chronic SDHs are more than 2 to 3 weeks old and are typically lower in attenuation than brain on CT.
- A history of trauma may be absent.
- Predisposing factors are older age, anticoagulant therapy, long-term hemodialysis, thrombocytopenia, and alcoholism.
- Ventricular decompression for hydrocephalus may cause SDHs.
- Acute-on-chronic SDHs develop from repeated hemorrhage into previous subdural collections.
- Fluid-blood levels are seen when sedimented fresh blood gravitates dependently and the proteinaceous fluid layers on top.

### ■ Other Imaging Findings

- Magnetic resonance imaging:
  - This shows hematomas along the tentorium and falx that are more difficult to evaluate on axial CT images.
  - Blood products of different ages can also be characterized to better advantage.

### ✓ Pearls & ✗ Pitfalls

✓ As the distance between the cerebral cortex and the dura increases as a result of atrophy, small veins extending from the cortex to the dura (so-called bridging veins) become stretched and can be sheared by violent head motions, even if the head has not been struck by external objects.

✓ Membranes can form within a chronic SDH, producing multiple compartments that have different attenuation characteristics.

✗ Subacute SDH becomes increasingly isodense to gray matter and difficult to detect on CT. When bilateral isodense SDHs are present, the mass effects in the two hemispheres can be balanced, making detection even more difficult.

# Case 46

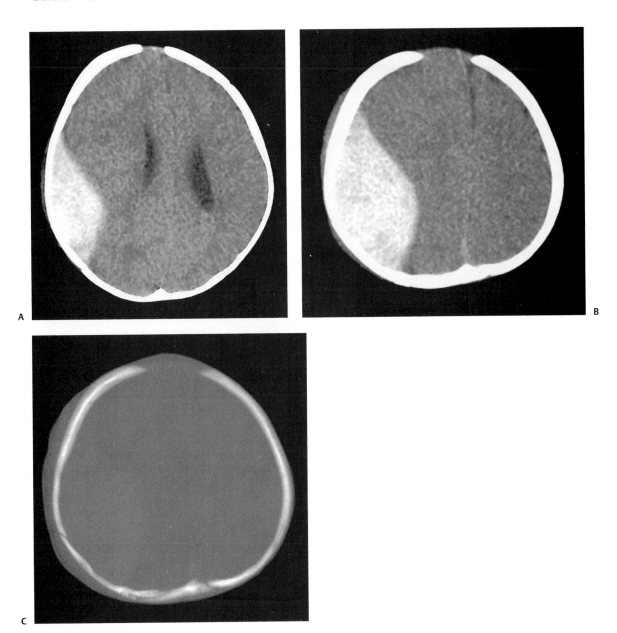

A

B

C

## ■ Clinical Presentation

A 7-month-old child after a fall.

## ■ Imaging Findings

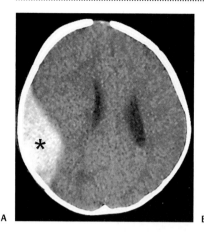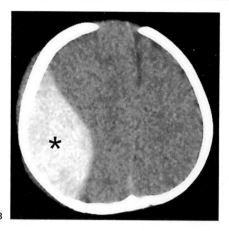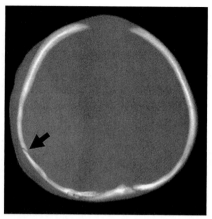

**(A,B)** Computed tomography (CT) scans of the brain demonstrate a lentiform collection of blood in the right frontoparietal convexity (*asterisk*). **(C)** Bone windows demonstrate a linear nondisplaced fracture in the right parietal bone (*arrow*).

## ■ Differential Diagnosis

- **Epidural hematoma (EDH):** This is a biconvex, hyperdense extra-axial fluid collection. There is adjacent skull fracture in 90% of cases. On occasion, subdural and epidural hematomas contain alternating crescent-shaped regions of various densities that produce a "swirled" appearance, considered an indication of active hemorrhage.
- *Subdural hematoma:* This is a crescentic, hyperdense collection between the arachnoid and dural membranes. There is displacement of the cortex away from the inner table. There is midline shift with compression of the ipsilateral lateral ventricle and dilatation of the contralateral ventricle.
- *Meningioma:* This dura-based tumor is isoattenuating to slightly hyperattenuating. Homogeneous and intense enhancement after the injection of iodinated contrast material is characteristic. Perilesional edema may be extensive. Hyperostosis and intratumoral calcifications may be present.

## ■ Essential Facts

- An EDH is a collection of blood between the inner skull table and the dura.
- There may be laceration of meningeal vessels, dural emissary veins, or sinuses.
- There is adjacent skull fracture in 90% of cases.
- Ninety-five percent are supratentorial.
- EDHs in the posterior fossa are rare and associated with higher morbidity and mortality than are supratentorial hematomas.

## ■ Other Imaging Findings

- Magnetic resonance imaging:
  - Hyperacute and chronic EDHs exhibit signal intensity similar to that of cerebrospinal fluid on T1 and T2-weighted images (WIs).
  - The acute EDH is isointense on T1WIs and iso- to hypointense on T2WIs.
  - Subacute and early chronic EDHs are hyperintense on T1- and T2WIs.

## ✓ Pearls & ✗ Pitfalls

- ✓ EDH does not cross cranial sutures, where the dura is tightly adherent.
- ✓ EDH may cross the falx or displace the dural venous sinuses from the inner table.
- ✓ Emergent surgical treatment is nearly always needed.
- ✗ EDH in the posterior fossa and along the floor of the anterior cranial fossa may be more difficult to visualize on CT.

# Case 47

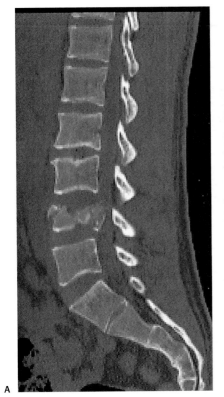

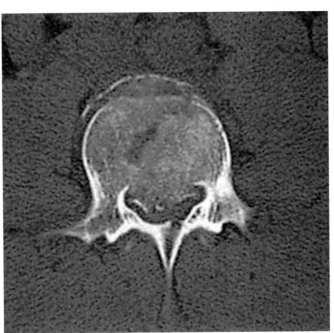

A                                                                                                 B

## Clinical Presentation

A woman with severe back pain after being in an automobile-pedestrian accident.

### Further Work-up

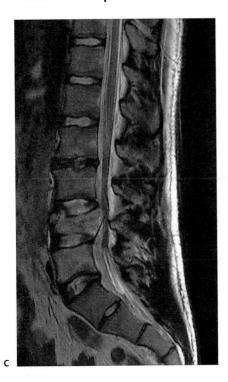

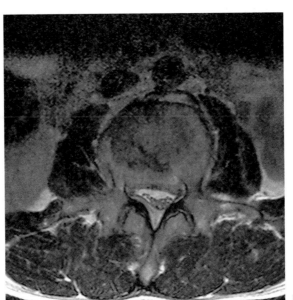

C                                                                                                 D

### ■ Imaging Findings

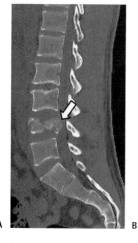
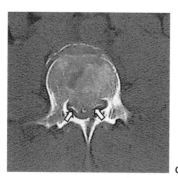
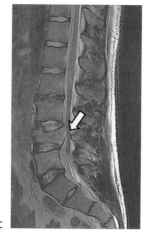
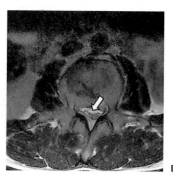

**(A)** Sagittal computed tomography (CT) scan of the lumbar spine shows a fracture of the L4 vertebral body involving all the walls, with retropulsion of fragments toward the spinal canal (*arrow*). **(B)** Axial CT scan of the lumbar spine shows a fracture of the L4 vertebral body involving all the walls, with retropulsion of fragments toward the spinal canal (*arrows*). There is also fracture of the posterior elements. **(C)** Sagittal T2-weighted image (WI) shows, in addition to the deformity of L4, bone marrow edema at L4 and L5. The narrowing of the canal and its effect on the cauda equina (*arrow*) are better demonstrated. **(D)** Axial T2WI shows flattening of the thecal sac (*arrow*) secondary to stenosis caused by the posteriorly displaced fracture fragments.

### ■ Differential Diagnosis

- **Burst fracture:** This is a compression fracture in which the entire vertebral body breaks. It results from axial loading that is most often secondary to motor vehicle accidents and falls. The axial load drives the intervertebral disk into the vertebral body below.
- *Pathologic fracture:* This occurs in a bone weakened as a result of neoplasm (multiple myeloma, metastatic bone disease). Fractures above the T7 level, fractures that present with a soft-tissue mass or osseous destruction, and fractures of the posterior part of the vertebral body are most likely to have a malignant etiology.
- *Vertebral fracture due to osteomalacia:* Osteomalacia causes bone softening and consequent biconcave deformity of the end plates ("codfish" vertebrae). In adulthood, these fractures resemble those found in osteoporosis. Usually, osseous deformities at other sites of the skeleton (e.g., protrusion acetabuli, pseudofractures [Looser zones] in the pelvis, and bone deformities) are also identified.

### ■ Essential Facts

- Depending on the mechanism of injury, predictable patterns of fracture-dislocation are identified (hyperflexion, hyperflexion-rotation, hyperextension, hyperextension-rotation, vertical compression, or lateral flexion).
- In the lower cervical segment of C3-C7 and in the thoraco-lumbar spine, support is provided by three columns:
  - Anterior column: the anterior vertebral bodies, anterior annulus fibrosus, and anterior longitudinal ligaments
  - Middle column: posterior vertebral bodies, posterior longitudinal ligaments, and posterior annulus fibrosus
  - Posterior column: posterior bony elements, ligamenta flava, and posterior ligaments
- The integrity of the middle column is the most crucial to spinal stability.

### ■ Other Imaging Findings

- Multidetector computed tomography (MDCT) is the modality of choice for the initial evaluation of bone injuries after blunt trauma to the cervical spine.
- When MDCT is not available, plain film remains the initial imaging modality. However, in patients who have unexplained focal pain, neurologic deficit with negative plain films, unexplained soft-tissue swelling, or abnormal plain films, additional evaluation with MDCT is indicated.
- Magnetic resonance imaging will show soft-tissue injury, spinal cord injury, intervertebral disk and ligament injury, and vascular injury.

### ✓ Pearls & ✗ Pitfalls

- ✓ Elderly patients usually have significant osteoporosis and degenerative bone disease.
- ✓ These patients may experience a significant fracture from a relatively minor trauma.
- ✓ They also may have pathologic fractures.
- ✗ Spinal cord injury in infants and young children often occurs without evidence of fracture or dislocation because of the inherent elasticity of their vertebral column, which makes the cord vulnerable to injury.
- ✗ Patients who have spinal cord injury without radiographic abnormality often have a poor long-term prognosis.

# Case 48

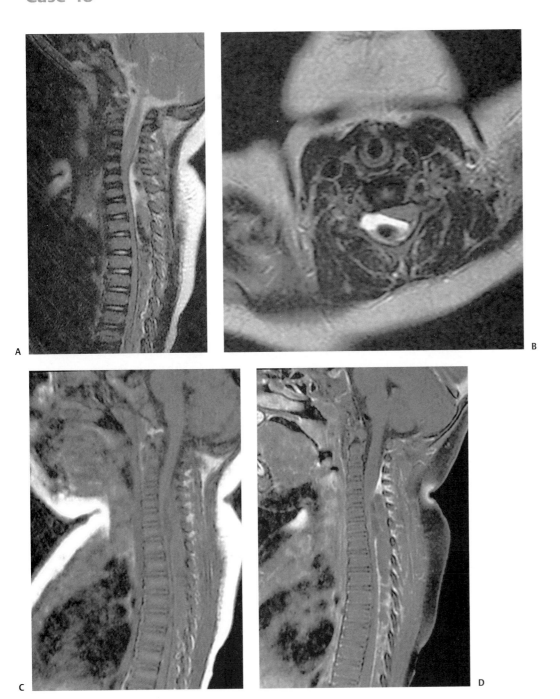

A

B

C

D

## Clinical Presentation

A 1-year-old with the sudden onset of bilateral lower extremity weakness.

### ▨ Imaging Findings

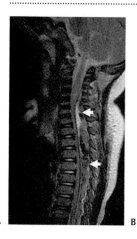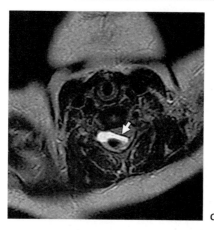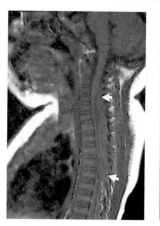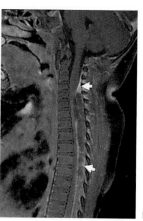

A   B   C   D

**(A)** Sagittal T2-weighted image (WI) shows a biconcave collection in the lower cervical and upper thoracic dorsal epidural space (*arrows*) with heterogeneous signal and areas of low signal. **(B)** In this axial image, the dura is visualized as a linear structure with low signal (*arrow*) between the anteriorly located cord and the hematoma. Note the compressive effect on the cord, which does not show edema. **(C,D)** Sagittal T1WIs, pre- and postcontrast administration, show scattered linear areas of enhancement (*arrows*) within and at the periphery of the collection.

### ▨ Differential Diagnosis

- ***Epidural hematoma (EDH):*** EDH is an extra-axial collection of blood with heterogeneous signal intensity and a biconvex shape. Displacement of the dura toward the cord confirms the epidural location of the lesion.
- *Epidural abscess:* This is an expanding suppurative infection in the spinal epidural space. Epidural abscesses impinge on the spinal cord and may cause vascular compromise and infarction. The thoracic spine is more frequently involved.
- *Epidural metastasis:* This is usually associated with vertebral infiltration and pathologic fracture. It spares the disk.

### ▨ Essential Facts

- Spinal EDH:
  - Etiology: trauma, anticoagulation therapy, vascular anomalies, spinal epidural procedures, spinal surgery, spontaneous
  - Symptoms: severe localized back pain with delayed radicular radiation that may mimic disk herniation
  - Treatment: emergency evacuation

### ▨ Other Imaging Findings

- Radiography and computed tomography (CT) are helpful in patients with a history of acute trauma to evaluate associated fractures or dislocation preoperatively and to assess the placement of instrumentation postoperatively.

- CT-myelography is indicated in patients who have spinal instrumentation, especially because the details of the spinal canal are often obscured by metal artifacts on magnetic resonance imaging (MRI). The hematoma is demonstrated as a biconvex filling defect in the spinal canal that usually extends over more than two vertebral levels.
- MRI:
  - Sagittal MRI usually shows the biconvex hematoma in the dorsal epidural space, with well-defined contours and tapering of the superior and inferior margins.
  - The hematomas show signal intensity that varies over time.
  - Displaced dura on sagittal or axial MRI is an important finding that indicates the epidural location of the hematoma.
  - The hematoma may demonstrate contrast enhancement.

### ✓ Pearls & ✗ Pitfalls

- ✓ Hyperintense cord lesions, which represent edema, compression myelopathy, contusion injury, or infarction, decrease the possibility of neurologic recovery.
- ✓ The cord involvement is better evaluated on axial than on sagittal images, particularly when the lesion is off the midline.
- ✗ Contrast enhancement of the cord parenchyma can be present and should not be misinterpreted as a neoplastic or an inflammatory cord lesion.

# Case 49

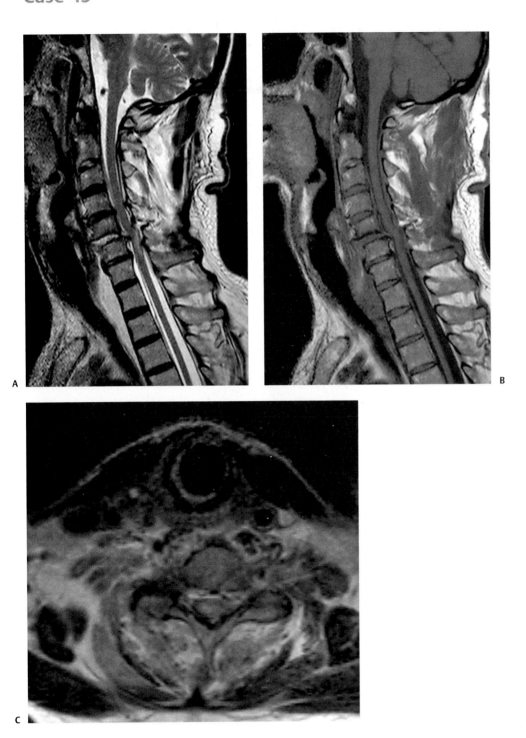

A

B

C

## ▦ Clinical Presentation

A 37-year-old woman presenting with motor and sensory disturbances in the arms and legs after a motor vehicle accident.

■ **Imaging Findings**

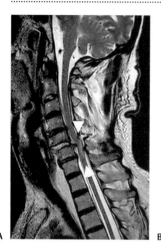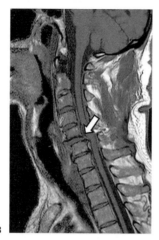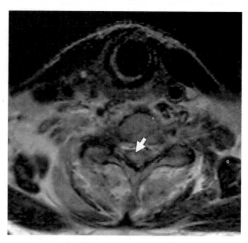

A                        B                                              C

**(A)** Sagittal T2-weighted image (WI) shows subluxation and disk edema at C5–C6 with posterior osteophytes. Narrowing of the canal and edema of the cord (*between arrowheads*) are noted. **(B)** Sagittal T1WI shows subluxation and disk widening at C5–C6 (*arrow*). There are posterior osteophytes. **(C)** Note the central cord edema on the axial T2WI (*arrow*). No cord hemorrhage is demonstrated.

■ **Differential Diagnosis**

- *Cord contusion:* Contusions tend to be severe in patients with degenerative changes. Magnetic resonance imaging (MRI) demonstrates increased cord signal and cord expansion.
- *Wallerian degeneration of the cord:* This develops in the subacute phase (about 1 month) after spinal cord injury. MRI reveals hyperintense signal on T2WIs in the white matter tracts above (dorsal columns) and below (lateral columns) the level of the injury.
- *Cord infarction:* This presents as the acute onset of myelopathy and is often heralded by sudden and severe back pain, which may radiate caudally. MRI shows a central cord lesion on the axial T2WIs. Causes include arteritis, embolism, aortic dissection, aortic surgery, decompression sickness, abdominal surgery, vertebral fracture, and disk herniation.

■ **Essential Facts**

- Cord contusions are classified clinically as complete lesions (loss of motor and sensory function at the injured level and distally) or incomplete lesions (central cord syndrome, anterior cord syndrome, Brown-Séquard syndrome, conus medullaris syndrome, cauda equina syndrome).
- Trauma to the spinal cord involves either true cord injury or compression with secondary cord damage.
- Acute MRI findings:
  - Transection
  - Intramedullary hemorrhage that is usually associated with a clinically complete and irreversible spinal cord injury

  - Contusion
  - Edema
  - Ligamentous injuries, muscular lesions, facet joint dislocations, and bone marrow edema
- Chronic MRI findings:
  - Syringomyelia: cystic degeneration of the injured spinal cord at or near the site of trauma
  - Progressive posttraumatic myelomalacic myelopathy, which may occur at 2 months and up to 30 years following injury
  - Spinal cord atrophy

■ **Other Imaging Findings**

- Although plain radiography still has a role in spinal cord trauma, particularly cervical spinal cord trauma, it has largely been replaced by multislice computed tomography.
- The multislice coronal and sagittal reconstructions often reveal more than plain radiographs do, and fractures and joint dislocations can be detected accurately.

✓ **Pearls & ✗ Pitfalls**

✓ Spinal cord injury without radiographic abnormality (SCIWORA) is well-known in the pediatric population.

✓ It is a consequence of the inherent elasticity of the vertebral column in infants and young children, which makes the pediatric spine exceedingly vulnerable to deforming forces.

✗ In the chronic stage of cervical injuries, intramedullary cysts should be differentiated from expected "static" myelomalacia, which has a less well-defined border and is not progressive.

# Case 50

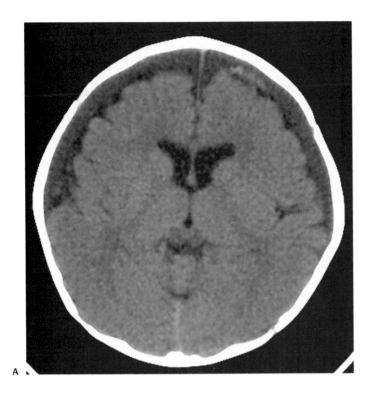

A

## Clinical Presentation

A 7-month-old child with a history of vomiting. Retinal hemorrhages were found at the clinical examination.

## Further Work-up

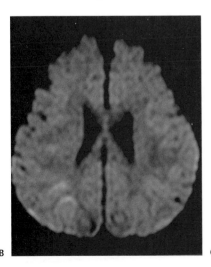

B

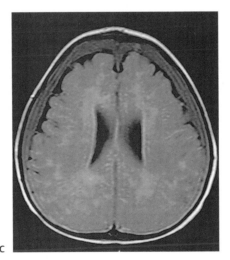

C

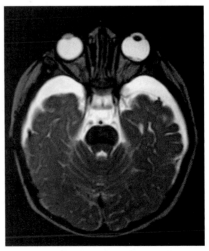

D

## Imaging Findings

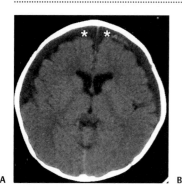 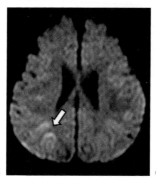 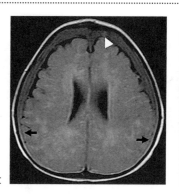 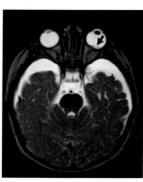

**(A)** Computed tomography (CT) of the brain demonstrates subdural collections in both frontal convexities, with mixed attenuation (*asterisks*). **(B)** Diffusion-weighted magnetic resonance imaging (MRI) shows restricted diffusion in the right parietal subcortical white matter (*arrow*). **(C)** Axial fluid-attenuated inversion recovery image shows hematocrit effect, with blood elements layering in the dependant portion of the collection (*arrows*) and focal areas of high signal within the subdural space anteriorly, consistent with acute blood (*arrowhead*). **(D)** Note the presence of retinal hemorrhages in the posterior pole of the left globe (*arrow*).

## Differential Diagnosis

- *Nonaccidental head injury (NAHI):* NAHI should be suspected in an infant or young child who presents with no history of injury; with a discrepancy between the explanation and nature of the lesions; with injuries of different ages or multiple injuries; with associated retinal hemorrhages; or with a change or inconsistency in the history, delayed medical care, repeated injuries, or evidence of overall poor care.
- *Benign external hydrocephalus with spontaneous hemorrhage:* Prominent subarachnoid spaces in infants are secondary to insufficient resorption of cerebrospinal fluid (CSF) as a result of immature arachnoid villi. These should be of the same density/intensity as CSF on CT and MRI. The condition predisposes infants to subdural hematoma (SDH), which may be spontaneous or associated with trauma of any type.
- *Subdural hygroma:* This is a CSF collection secondary to traumatic arachnoid tears. Attenuation and signal intensity are similar to those of CSF. Blood vessels crossing through the extra-axial collection will help differentiate subdural hygromas from chronic SDHs.

## Essential Facts

- NAHI is the leading cause of morbidity and mortality in abused children.
- NAHI occurs in ~12% of physically abused children.
- It accounts for 80% of deaths from head injury in children younger than 2 years of age.
- Clinical presentation: the triad of subdural hemorrhage, retinal hemorrhage, and encephalopathy (i.e., diffuse axonal injury) occurs in the context of an inappropriate or inconsistent history and is commonly accompanied by other apparently inflicted injuries.

- Spectrum of injuries:
  - Skull fracture (multiple or complex fractures, bilateral fractures, and fractures that cross suture lines or involve more than one bone are more suspicious)
  - SDH
  - Shearing injury
  - Cerebral contusions
  - Brain swelling
  - Cerebral infarction (caused by shaking, strangulation, smothering)
  - Chronic injuries (chronic SDH, communicating hydrocephalus, atrophy, or encephalomalacia)

## Other Imaging Findings

- Imaging evaluation includes CT, a radiographic or radionuclide skeletal survey, MRI, and serial imaging in some cases.
- Nonhead injuries associated with non-accidental trauma include rib fracture, metaphyseal fracture, vertebral compression fracture, and small-bowel hematoma and laceration.

## ✓ Pearls & ✗ Pitfalls

- ✓ Skull fractures are not rare in household trauma but rarely present with significant underlying brain injury (with the exception of epidural hematoma).
- ✓ Soft-tissue swelling may be absent, even in acute skull fracture; thus, a lack of swelling should not be construed as evidence that the fracture is subacute.
- ✗ Retinal hemorrhages have been reported with accidental trauma, resuscitation, increased intracranial pressure, increased venous pressure, subarachnoid hemorrhage, sepsis, coagulopathy, certain metabolic disorders, systemic hypertension, and other conditions, and are therefore not specific for NAHI.

# Case 51

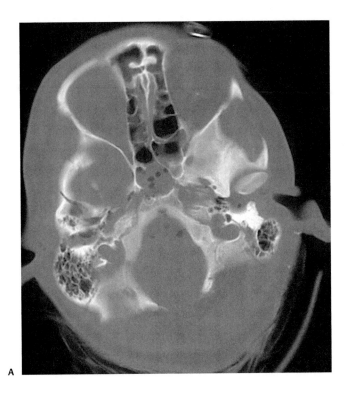

A

## ■ Clinical Presentation

A 36-year-old woman injured in a motor vehicle collision.

## Further Work-up

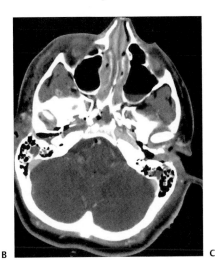

B

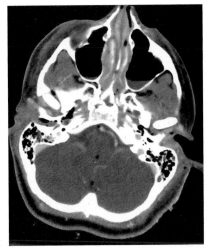

C

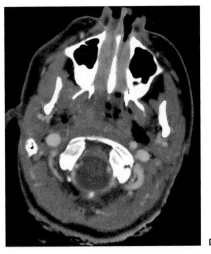

D

### ■ Imaging Findings

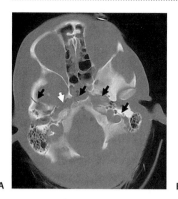 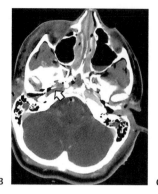 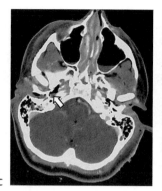 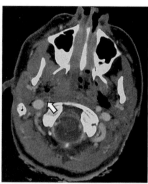

A                    B                    C                    D

**(A)** Computed tomography (CT) of the brain with bone windows shows a complex fracture of the skull base involving the sphenoid and temporal bones (*black arrows*) and compromise of the anterolateral wall of the right carotid canal (*white arrow*). **(B)** Axial image from a CT angiogram (CTA) of the brain shows absent opacification of the petrous right internal carotid artery (ICA) secondary to traumatic vascular injury (*arrow*). **(C)** Axial image from a CTA of the brain shows absent opacification of the petrous right ICA secondary to traumatic vascular injury (*arrow*). Pneumocephalus and neck emphysema are also noted. **(D)** Axial CTA at the level of C1 shows absent flow in the right ICA secondary to traumatic vascular injury (*arrow*). Pneumocephalus and neck emphysema are also noted.

### ■ Differential Diagnosis

- **Skull base fracture with arterial transection:** Direct injury to the vessel is caused by the displaced bone fragments. Symptoms of stroke may be masked by the brain injuries.
- *Extracranial carotid dissection:* This is a posttraumatic intimal tear that commonly affects the distal ICA. Some tears probably heal spontaneously, but others lead to dissection for a variable distance, with or without pseudoaneurysm formation, and some thrombose.
- *Embolic occlusion of the ICA:* The appearance of the vessels would be similar, but this diagnosis is less likely in the setting of skull base fractures.

### ■ Essential Facts

- Because of the complex anatomic relationships of the skull base, fractures may damage critical neighboring structures, including cranial nerves, the ICA, and the cavernous sinus.
- Complications:
  - Vascular injuries: carotid-cavernous fistula, pseudoaneurysm, dissection, sinus thrombosis
  - Cerebrospinal fluid (CSF) fistula and infection
  - Cranial nerve injury
  - Central nervous system injury: contusions, extra-axial hemorrhages, brainstem infarctions, and posterior pituitary dysfunction in the form of diabetes insipidus

### ■ Other Imaging Findings

- CTA is used to identify potentially treatable vascular injuries.
- For the localization of CSF fistulas, high-resolution CT with or without cisternography, heavily T2-weighted coronal magnetic resonance (MR) imaging, gadolinium-enhanced MR cisternography, or intrathecal radioisotope studies have been proposed.

### ✓ Pearls & ✗ Pitfalls

- ✓ Frontal sinus fractures may lead to cosmetic deformity, CSF fistula, chronic meningitis, and mucocele. Sinus cranialization may be necessary to prevent CSF leak and meningitis.
- ✓ Temporal bone fractures may cause damage of the facial nerve, labyrinthine fistula, conductive or sensorineural hearing loss, CSF leak, or cephalocele.
- ✗ Air in the cavernous sinuses may be the result of embolism from intravenous access and does not always indicate basilar skull fracture.

# Case 52

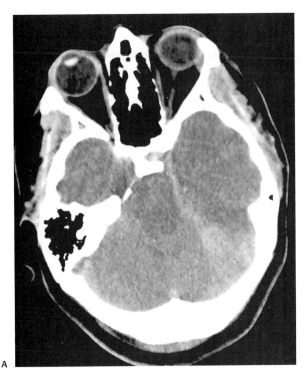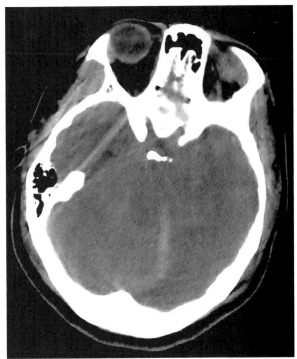

A | B

## ■ Clinical Presentation

A 26-year-old who was involved in a car accident and is now comatose.

## Further Work-up

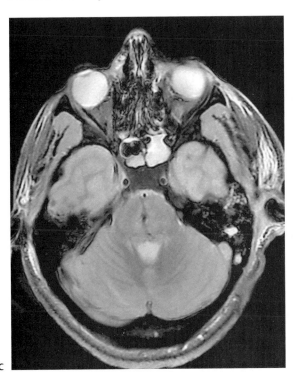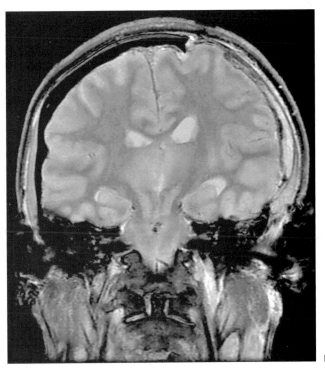

C | D

### ■ Imaging Findings

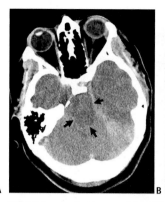
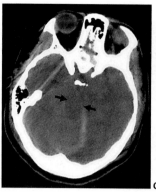
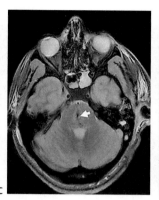
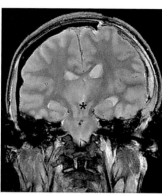

A B C D

**(A)** Axial computed tomography (CT) of the brain shows signs of cerebral edema, with low attenuation of the brain and loss of distinction between gray and white matter. Effacement of the basal cisterns (*arrows*) and deformity of the midbrain are evident. **(B)** Axial CT demonstrates effacement of the perimesencephalic cistern (*arrows*) and deformity of the midbrain, with reduced transverse diameter and elongation in the anteroposterior direction. Note a subdural hematoma over the left tentorium. **(C)** Axial gradient-echo T2*-weighted image (WI) reveals petechial hemorrhages in the central pons (*arrow*). **(D)** Coronal T2WI shows downward displacement of the thalami and midbrain (*asterisk*). The pontine hemorrhages are again demonstrated.

### ■ Differential Diagnosis

- **Duret hemorrhages:** Duret hemorrhages are brainstem hemorrhages that develop as a consequence of downward trans-tentorial herniation. Magnetic resonance imaging (MRI) findings of descending trans-tentorial herniation include lower position of the brainstem, effacement of the basal cisterns, flattening of the pons against the clivus, and inferoposterior displacement of the quadrigeminal plate.
- *Interpeduncular subarachnoid hemorrhage:* This is usually an early occurrence in trauma patients and can be mistaken for parenchymal hemorrhage.
- *Shearing injury:* This is characterized by multiple small hemorrhages in the deep white matter, including the corpus callosum and brainstem. In the pons, it may appear identical to and coexist with Duret hemorrhages.

### ■ Essential Facts

- Descending trans-tentorial herniation consists of caudal descent of brain tissue through the tentorial incisura and occurs mainly in response to mass effect in the frontal, parietal, and occipital lobes.
- The lower brainstem is made less mobile by the upper cervical dentate ligaments. Longitudinal compression of the upper brainstem against the unyielding medulla leads to buckling of the brainstem and further compression of the midbrain tegmentum.

- Stretching and shearing of the perforating branches of the basilar artery occur, resulting in ischemia and hemorrhage within the brainstem, called Duret hemorrhage.
- The clinical consequences of progressive central herniation are oculomotor paresis, progressive alteration of consciousness, decerebrate rigidity, coma, and death.

### ✓ Pearls & ✗ Pitfalls

✓ Downward descent of the brain may be secondary to intracranial hypotension, which is caused by either an iatrogenic or a spontaneous cerebrospinal fluid leak.

✓ There may be pachymeningeal venous engorgement and edema, downward descent of the brain, and descending central trans-tentorial or tonsillar herniation.

✗ Diffuse cerebral edema results in symmetric abnormalities on CT and MRI that may be overlooked.

✗ The distortion of the brainstem caused by downward trans-tentorial herniation may mimic a Chiari type II malformation.

# Case 53

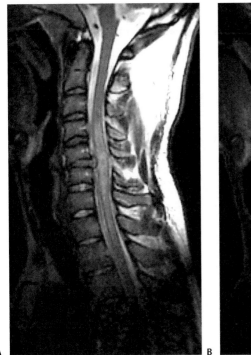
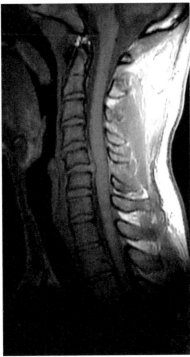
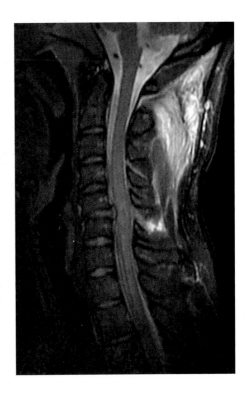

A

B

C

## Clinical Presentation

A 21-year-old woman who fell on her head during gymnastics practice.

## Further Work-up

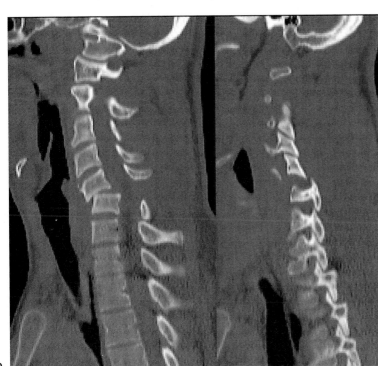

D

■ **Imaging Findings**

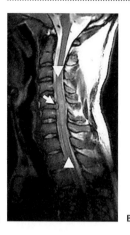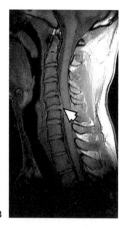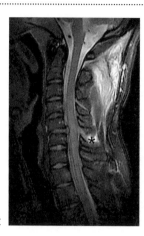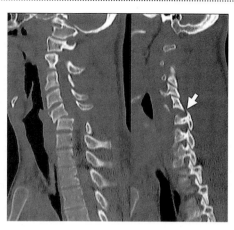

A  B  C  D

**(A)** Sagittal T2-weighted image (WI) demonstrates a disk protrusion (*arrow*) at C5-C6 impinging on the spinal cord, which demonstrates significant edema (*between arrowheads*). **(B)** Sagittal T1WI shows widening of the intervertebral space posteriorly (*arrowhead*). **(C)** Fat-suppressed sagittal T2WI shows disruption of the C5-C6 interspinous ligament with widening and edema (*asterisk*). There is also edema of the dorsal paraspinal soft tissues in the upper cervical region. **(D)** Sagittal and parasagittal reformatted images of a computed tomography (CT) scan obtained 12 hours earlier, before traction, show anterior translation of C5 on C6 secondary to facet dislocation (*arrow*), which was bilateral.

■ **Differential Diagnosis**

• **Traumatic disk herniation and cord contusion:** Traumatic injuries can be suspected when the disk has a high signal on T2WIs. Also, concomitant traumatic vertebral body injuries and/or ligamentous injuries may be suggestive of traumatic disk lesions.
• *Cord contusion secondary to chronic degenerative disk disease:* In some cases, it may not be possible to determine if the disk herniation was present before the injury or is posttraumatic in nature. Patients with degenerative spinal stenosis are at higher risk for cord contusion.
• *Epidural hematoma:* The signal intensity of an acute epidural hematoma may be similar to that of the herniated disk material. The shape of the herniated disk and its connection with the native disk may help to differentiate them.

■ **Essential Facts**

• Traumatic disk herniation is commonly caused by distraction and shearing in sudden extension, but it also occurs in flexion injuries.
• Cervical disk herniations are seen in 54 to 80% of patients who have joint facet dislocation.
• High signal intensity seen horizontally through a disk (involving the nucleus and annulus on a T2WI) is highly suggestive of disk and annulus disruption.

■ **Other Imaging Findings**

• CT will assess the bone and the articular alignment but is insensitive for the evaluation of soft-tissue injuries in the spine.
• Magnetic resonance imaging is the modality of choice for the evaluation of cord injuries and disruption of the disks and ligaments.

✓ **Pearls & ✗ Pitfalls**

✓ The integrity of the diskoligamental complex (DLC) is thought to be directly proportional to spinal stability after cervical spine trauma.
✓ The components of the DLC are the intervertebral disk, anterior and posterior longitudinal ligaments, ligamenta flava, interspinous and supraspinous ligaments, and facet capsules.
✗ Traumatic and nontraumatic disk herniations can be similar in appearance.

# Case 54

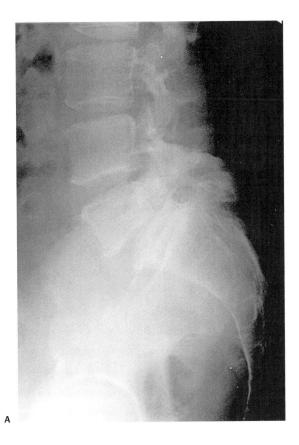

A

## Clinical Presentation

A 58-year-old man with left lumbar radiculopathy.

## Further Work-up

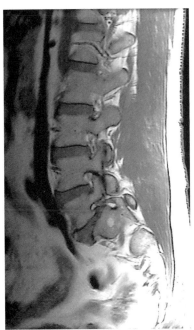

B

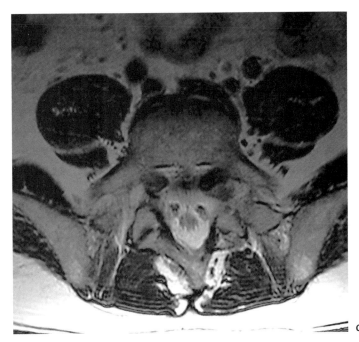

C

### ■ Imaging Findings

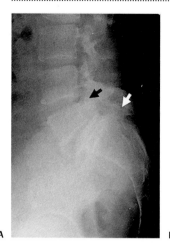
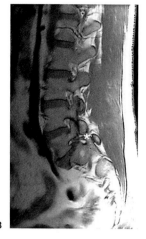
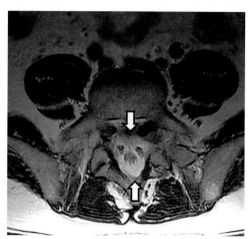

**(A)** Lateral radiograph of the lumbar spine demonstrates anterior slippage of L5 on S1. There is a gap between the superior *(black arrow)* and inferior *(white arrow)* facets of L5. **(B)** Sagittal T1-weighted image (WI) confirms anterior displacement of L5 with respect to S1, with a fat-filled gap between the superior and inferior facets of L5 *(asterisk)*. **(C)** Axial T1WI shows elongation of the anteroposterior diameter of the spinal canal secondary to anterolisthesis *(arrows)*.

### ■ Differential Diagnosis

• **Spondylolysis with spondylolisthesis:** This is a focal interruption of the pars interarticularis. This interruption causes forward slippage of the superior vertebral body (spondylolisthesis). If significant anterolisthesis of the vertebral body is present, a fat-filled gap between the pars fragments can sometimes be appreciated.

• *Degenerative lumbar spondylolisthesis:* Osteoarthritis of the facet joints is characterized by thinning of the cartilage, sclerotic changes in the subchondral bone, osteophyte formation, synovial inflammation, and capsular ligament laxity. In more severe forms of the process, osteoarthritis of a facet joint may lead to hypermobility of the facet joint and then to a spondylolisthesis. Most cases of degenerative spondylolisthesis occur at the L4-L5 level.

• *Posttraumatic spondylolisthesis:* This is associated with acute fracture of a posterior element (pedicle, lamina, or facets) other than the pars interarticularis.

### ■ Essential Facts

• Spondylolysis is a bone defect in the pars interarticularis.
• It results from repeated microfractures and elongation of a congenitally weakened pars, usually first becoming radiographically visible in late childhood or adolescence.
• Typically, the pars defects remain bridged by fibrocartilage but may form a pseudojoint.
• Occasionally, healing and bone union occur, a phenomenon likely accounting for many of the 10 to 15% of cases with unilateral defects.
• The L5 vertebra is involved in 90 to 95% of patients.
• Men are affected two to four times more often than women.

• Approximately 25% of patients with lumbar spondylolysis eventually have significant lower back pain or sciatica, caused by muscular and ligamentous strain, spinal or foraminal stenosis, facet degeneration, and associated disk degeneration or herniation.

### ■ Other Imaging Findings

• Radiographs allow visualization and grading of spondylolisthesis but may not always reveal spondylolysis. Dynamic studies in flexion and extension can aid the diagnosis. The "Scotty dog with a broken neck" can be seen on oblique films in patients who have a classic spondylolysis.
• Computed tomography allows better visualization of the spondylolytic defect.
• MRI may visualize edema in the marrow around the site of an acute spondylolytic defect and is helpful for identifying nerve root compression resulting from foraminal or central canal stenosis.

### ✓ Pearls & ✗ Pitfalls

✓ Bilateral spondylolysis may result in a large degree of slippage, whereas degenerative facet arthropathy typically results in a lesser degree of displacement.
✓ Degenerative spondylolisthesis is seen most commonly at the L4-L5 level.
✗ Sclerosis of the pars and partial volume averaging of adjacent facet arthropathy can produce a focal signal loss in the pars that is nearly indistinguishable from that seen in spondylolysis on MRI.

# Case 55

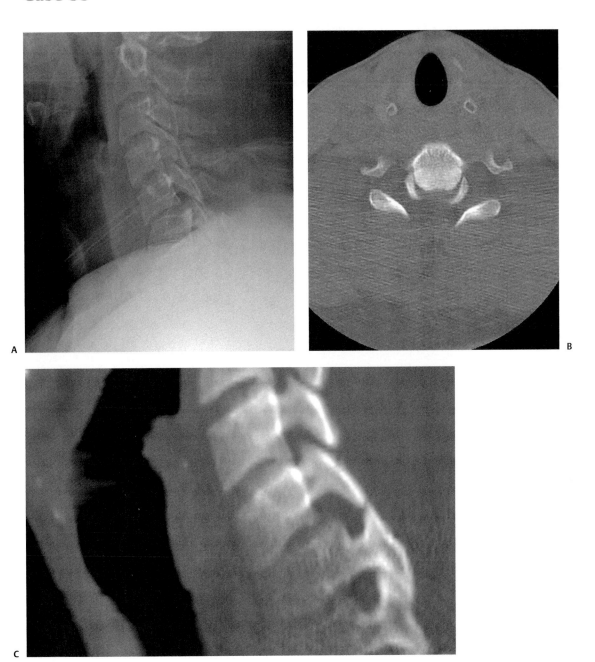

## ■ Clinical Presentation

A 32-year-old with neck pain and lower leg numbness after a car accident.

### ■ Imaging Findings

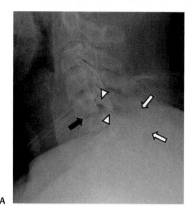
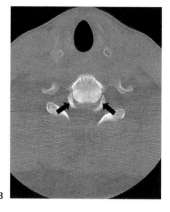
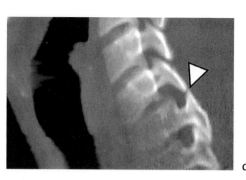

A        B        C

**(A)** Lateral radiograph of the cervical spine shows "fanning" of the spinous process at the C5-C6 level (*white arrows*), widening and displacement of the joint facets (*arrowheads*), wedging of the intervertebral space (*black arrow*), and fracture of the C5 spinous process. The prevertebral soft tissues are thickened at this level. **(B)** Axial computed tomography (CT) of the cervical spine at C5-C6 shows posterior displacement of the uncovertebral joints of C6 (*arrows*). **(C)** Reformatted CT maximum-intensity projection image shows the perched facet joint (*arrowhead*).

### ■ Differential Diagnosis

- ***Anterior subluxation in hyperflexion sprain of the cervical spine:*** Hyperflexion injuries are associated with localized kyphotic angulation; anterior displacement or rotation; wedge narrowing of the vertebral disk space (widened posteriorly); anterior displacement of the inferior facets, which can appear widened, perched, or completely "locked"; "fanning" of the interspinous space; and anterior pillar fracture.
- *Hyperextension injury to the cervical spine:* This injury can be associated with fracture of the anterior arch of the atlas, compression fracture of the posterior arch of the atlas, fractures of the dens, traumatic spondylolisthesis of C2 (hangman's fracture), tear drop fracture, laminar fracture, and wedging of the intervertebral joint space (widened anteriorly).
- *Flexion and rotation injury of the cervical spine:* This is associated with laminar fractures, unilateral perched facet, rotational subluxation of the vertebral bodies, and misalignment of the spinous processes.

### ■ Essential Facts

- Hyperflexion of the cervical spine causes a disruption of the posterior ligaments.
- There is a disruption of the joint facet capsule with anterior displacement of the inferior joint facets. The inferior articular process of the vertebra above may lie atop (perched) or anterior to (locked) the superior articular process of the vertebra below.

### ■ Other Imaging Findings

- CT is helpful for the evaluation of fractures and displacements of the facets joints. It also helps to identify fracture fragments.
- Ligamentous injuries are better seen on magnetic resonance imaging (MRI). A T2-weighted fat-saturated sequence is the sequence of choice. MRI is recommended to evaluate the spinal cord; cord edema will show increased signal on the T2-weighted image.
- The uncovered articular surfaces of a displaced zygapophyseal joint have been described as the "naked facet" sign.

### ✓ Pearls & ✗ Pitfalls

- ✓ MRI is helpful to detect soft-tissue and cervical cord injuries.
- ✓ Rotation in the lateral view of the cervical spine can obscure facet joint displacements.
- ✓ The vertebral arteries run in the transverse foramen of the cervical spine; assessment for vascular injury is necessary.
- ✗ Controversy exists in the literature on how appropriate the term *locked facet* is because it can suggest stability of a very unstable injury.

# Case 56

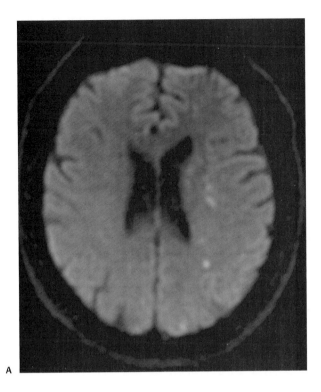

A

## Clinical Presentation

A 55-year-old man with the sudden onset of right-sided weakness and neck pain.

## Further Work-up

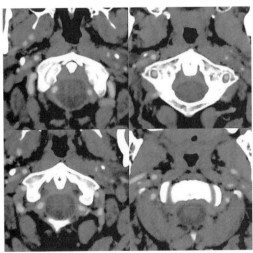

B

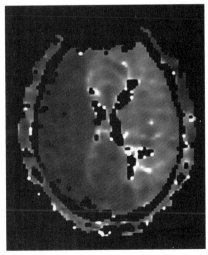

C

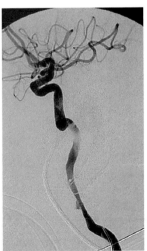

D

### ■ Imaging Findings

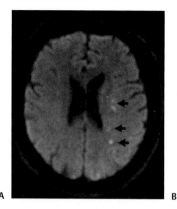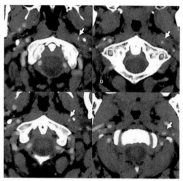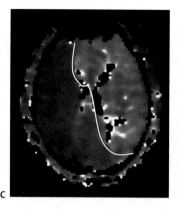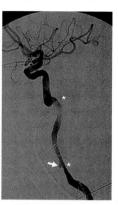

A   B   C   D

**(A)** Axial diffusion-weighted image (WI) demonstrates multiple punctate foci of restriction in the left centrum semiovale, consistent with acute watershed infarcts (*arrows*). **(B)** Serial axial images from a computed tomography (CT) angiogram show narrowing of the left internal carotid artery (ICA) with a rotating flat lumen (*arrows*). **(C)** CT perfusion time-to-peak image demonstrates delayed cerebral blood flow in the territory of both anterior cerebral arteries and the left middle cerebral artery (*delineated*). **(D)** Digital subtraction angiography shows dissection of the left ICA from its origin, with a long segment of narrowing (*between asterisks*) and a spiral configuration of the lumen. There is a pseudoaneurysm in the proximal aspect of the dissection (*arrow*).

### ■ Differential Diagnosis

- **Carotid dissection:** This is characterized by a tear in the intima of the vessel, which allows intraluminal blood to dissect along the layers of the vessel wall, or alternatively a direct hemorrhage from the vasa vasorum of the media into the arterial wall. Luminal narrowing or total occlusion occurs if the hematoma lies just beneath the intima. If the hematoma dissects just beneath the adventitia, a pseudoaneurysm forms. A false lumen occurs if blood reenters the true lumen. The false lumen may remain patent, resolve completely, or thrombose and cause narrowing of the true lumen.
- *Traumatic pseudoaneurysm:* Traumatic pseudoaneurysm is caused by a disruption in the continuity of the arterial wall. It is a periarterial hematoma contained by adjacent soft tissues. Subsequent encapsulation results in pseudoaneurysm formation. It may be associated with dissection.
- *Atherosclerosis:* Narrowing in atherosclerosis tends to occur in short segments, at vessel origins, or at sites of turbulent flow. It is usually bilateral. It may be associated with dissection. Ulceration in a plaque may mimic a pseudoaneurysm.

### ■ Essential Facts

- Carotid artery dissection may occur spontaneously or in association with external trauma or vasculopathy (fibromuscular dysplasia and other connective tissue diseases, such as Ehlers-Danlos syndrome type IV, Marfan syndrome, autosomal-dominant adult polycystic kidney disease, osteogenesis imperfecta type I, and cystic medial necrosis).
- The clinical presentation includes stroke, Horner syndrome, face or neck pain, cranial neuropathy, and pulsatile tinnitus.

- The thrombosed dissection lumen may become the source of distal embolization presenting as a transient ischemic attack or stroke.
- Common locations:
  - Cervical ICA 2 to 3 cm distal to the carotid bulb
  - Vertebral artery at the level of C1-C2
  - Involving multiple vessels

### ■ Other Imaging Findings

- Angiography: Features include double lumen and intimal flap, arterial stenosis, tapered end, string sign or flame shape, aneurysm formation, and arterial occlusion. Appearance evolves with time.
- Magnetic resonance imaging (MRI): A narrowed eccentric flow void is surrounded by a crescent-shaped area of hyperintensity expanding the vessel diameter. T1 hyperintense signal from mural hematoma.

### ✓ Pearls & ✗ Pitfalls

✓ An acute intramural hematoma can be hypointense on T2WIs and T1WIs and is therefore difficult to delineate from an area of flow void. The intramural hematoma may therefore be missed on MRI within the first 24 to 48 hours after an ICA dissection.

✗ MRI may demonstrate T1 hyperintense fat around the vessel, which can mimic an intramural hematoma; fat-suppression techniques are useful in such cases.

✗ In-flow phenomena, in the presence of slow blood flow, may mimic intraluminal thrombus. The signal abnormalities are located centrally within the flow void rather than peripherally. Homogeneity of the hyperintense signal on all slices associated with vessel expansion supports dissection rather than slow flow.

# Case 57

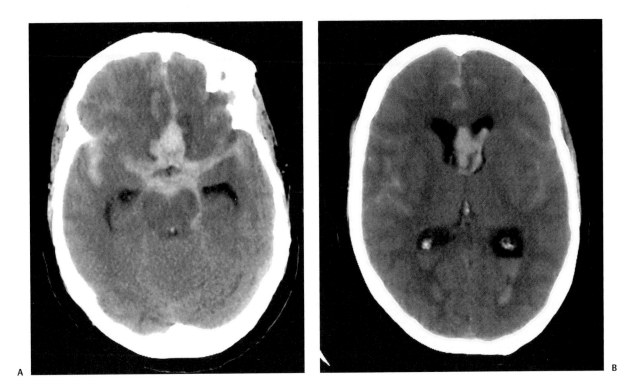

A                                                             B

## ■ Clinical Presentation

A young woman who has fallen from her own height after "the worst headache of her life."

## Further Work-up

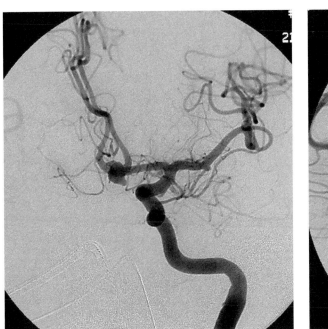

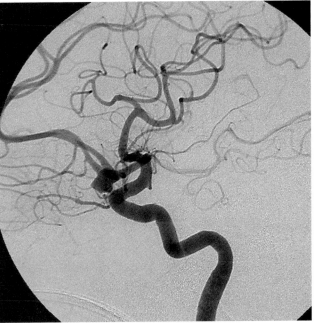

C                                                             D

■ **Imaging Findings**

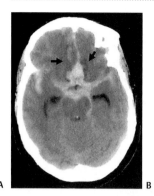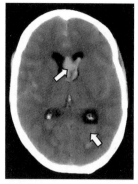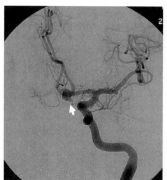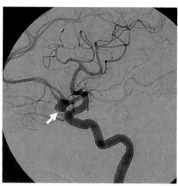

A   B   C   D

**(A)** Axial nonenhanced computed tomography (CT) shows subarachnoid hemorrhage (SAH) in the basal cisterns that is more prominent in the interhemispheric region. Areas of low attenuation in the gyri recti are noted, consistent with edema or ischemia (*arrows*). There is also intraventricular hemorrhage. **(B)** Axial nonenhanced CT shows SAH in the interhemispheric and sylvian regions. There is also intraventricular hemorrhage (*arrows*). **(C)** Oblique projection of a digital subtraction angiogram (DSA) of the left internal carotid artery (ICA) reveals a lobulated aneurysm in the anterior communicating artery (*arrow*). There is no narrowing of the vessels to suggest vasospasm. **(D)** Lateral projection of a DSA of the left ICA shows a lobulated aneurysm in the anterior communicating artery (*arrow*).

■ **Differential Diagnosis**

- **Ruptured cerebral aneurysm:** This causes SAH that is more extensive in the region of the aneurysm. It may also cause parenchymal or intraventricular hemorrhage.
- *Arteriovenous malformation (AVM):* This is a less common cause of SAH. Usually, parenchymal hemorrhage predominates. AVM may have calcifications and variable mass effect.
- *Traumatic SAH and frontal lobe contusion:* If a trauma patient presents with injuries that are disproportionate to the mechanism of trauma, another cause of subarachnoid and parenchymal hemorrhage should be sought.

■ **Essential Facts**

- Intracranial aneurysm is a localized pathologic dilatation of cerebral arteries.
- Types: saccular (berry aneurysm), dissecting, fusiform, infectious, traumatic, neoplastic
- Complications:
  - Rupture: SAH, parenchymal hematoma, hydrocephalus
  - Vasospasm: 4 to 5 days after rupture, secondary infarctions, leading cause of death
  - Mass effect: cranial nerve palsies, headache
  - Rebleeding: 50% within 6 months, 50% mortality
- Treatment options: endovascular coiling or craniotomy with clip ligation (clipping)

■ **Other Imaging Findings**

- CT angiography (CTA) is currently the first-choice examination in cases of SAH as it allows diagnosis of the aneurysm, analysis of its three-dimensional shape, and decisions regarding therapeutic choices.
- DSA is the gold standard and must be performed when the results of CTA and magnetic resonance angiography (MRA) are negative. If a four-vessel angiogram does not demonstrate the aneurysm, the external carotid arteries must be evaluated to exclude a dural fistula.
- MRA can be used to screen for unruptured aneurysms.

✓ **Pearls & ✗ Pitfalls**

- ✓ Aneurysms are multiple in 20% of cases.
- ✓ Useful signs to identify the one that bled:
  - Within the SAH
  - Largest aneurysm most likely to bleed
  - Most irregular aneurysm
  - Extravasation of contrast (rare)
  - Vasospasm adjacent to bleeding aneurysm
- ✓ There is an increased incidence of aneurysms in autosomal-dominant polycystic kidney disease, aortic coarctation, fibromuscular dysplasia, structural collagen disorders (Marfan syndrome, Ehlers-Danlos syndrome), neurofibromatosis type 1, and α1-antitrypsin deficiency.
- ✗ Do not mistake an infundibular dilatation of the posterior communicating artery for an aneurysm. It is round or conical in shape and 3 mm in maximum diameter. It has no aneurysmal neck, and the posterior communicating artery arises from its apex.

# Case 58

### ■ Imaging Findings

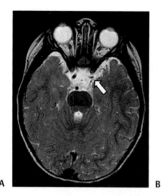 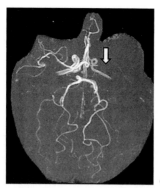 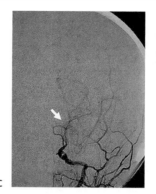 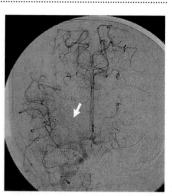

A                B                C                D

**(A)** Axial T2-weighted image (WI) of the brain shows narrowing of the left internal carotid artery (ICA) in the supraclinoid segment (*arrow*). **(B)** Magnetic resonance angiography (MRA) of the brain reveals narrowing of the left ICA with an absent flow-related signal in the left middle cerebral artery (MCA; *arrow*). There is also a paucity of branches of the right MCA. **(C)** Digital subtraction angiogram (DSA) of the left common carotid artery shows tapering and occlusion of the distal ICA. Prominent leptomeningeal collateral vessels are noted (*arrow*). **(D)** DSA of the left common carotid artery shows attenuation of the right MCA and both anterior cerebral arteries (ACAs). Hypertrophic leptomeningeal vessels give the appearance of a "puff of smoke" (*arrow*).

### ■ Differential Diagnosis

- **Moyamoya disease:** Moyamoya disease is characterized by occlusive changes in the distal ICAs or proximal ACAs or MCAs. Hypertrophy of the leptomeningeal collaterals results in a "puff of smoke" appearance on the angiogram.
- *Embolism of cardiac origin:* This causes occlusion of large or medium-size vessels with acute infarcts. It does not result in proliferation of the leptomeningeal vessels.
- *Fibromuscular dysplasia (FMD):* FMD causes multifocal concentric luminal narrowing alternating with areas of mural dilatation that are wider than the original lumen ("string of beads"). It may be associated with arterial dissection, intracranial aneurysms, and arteriovenous fistulas.

### ■ Essential Facts

- Moyamoya disease causes progressive occlusion of branches of the circle of Willis.
- The collateral network results in a "puff of smoke" appearance on angiograms.
- Moyamoya disease affects children in the first decade of life or adults in the third or fourth decade.
- Associated conditions are sickle cell anemia, Down syndrome, Fanconi anemia, and neurofibromatosis type 1. Moyamoya disease may also be associated with radiation therapy of the brain and may occur in families.

### ■ Other Imaging Findings

- MRA can delineate the occlusive changes and collateral networks.
- MR perfusion provides information regarding the cerebrovascular reserve that may aid in management.
- Cerebral angiography:
  - Stenosis or occlusion at the terminal portion of the ICA or the proximal portion of the ACAs or MCAs
  - Abnormal vascular networks in the vicinity of the occlusive or stenotic areas

### ✓ Pearls & ✗ Pitfalls

- ✓ The term *moyamoya disease* should be reserved for those cases in which the characteristic angiographic pattern is idiopathic.
- ✓ The term *moyamoya syndrome* is used when the underlying condition is known.
- ✗ Inadequate visualization of the flow void of the proximal vessels of the circle of Willis on axial T2WIs of the brain should raise the suspicion of occlusive changes.

# Case 59

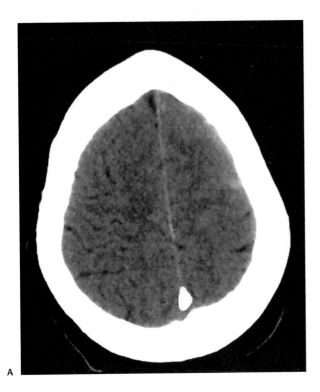

A

## Clinical Presentation

A 24-year-old postpartum patient with a history of headache.

## Further Work-up

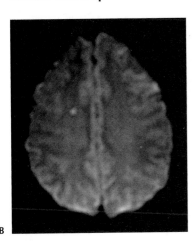

B

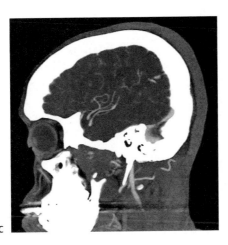

C

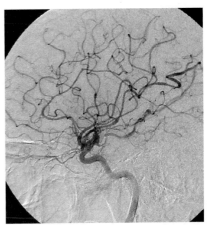

D

### ■ Imaging Findings

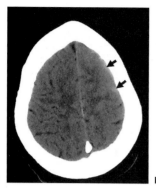 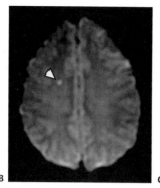 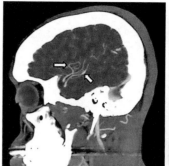 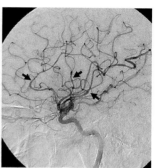

**(A)** Nonenhanced computed tomography (CT) of the brain demonstrates subarachnoid hemorrhage in the left frontal convexity (*arrows*). **(B)** Diffusion-weighted image shows a tiny focus of acute ischemia in the right centrum semiovale (*arrowhead*). Fluid-attenuated inversion recovery images (not shown) confirmed subarachnoid hemorrhage in the left convexity. **(C)** CT angiography, sagittal maximum-intensity-projection image, reveals a beaded appearance of some of the left middle cerebral artery (MCA) branches. **(D)** Lateral projection of a digital subtraction angiogram of the left internal carotid artery (ICA) shows multiple areas in the anterior cerebral artery and MCA branches with alternating segments of narrowing and dilatation (i.e., beading; *arrows*).

### ■ Differential Diagnosis

- **Central nervous system vasculitis:** This is characterized by inflammation and necrosis of blood vessel walls. Causes can be infectious or noninfectious. The condition can be attributed to immune complex deposition (polyarteritis nodosa, hypersensitivity vasculitis, collagen vascular disease) and can also be cell-mediated, as in giant cell arteritis (temporal arteritis, Takayasu arteritis, and granulomatous arteritis) or Wegener granulomatosis. Other causes include drug abuse, Kawasaki disease, neoplastic angiitis, and sarcoidosis.
- *Fibromuscular dysplasia:* Fibromuscular dysplasia is a nonatherosclerotic, noninflammatory arterial disease. It most commonly involves the renal and carotid arteries. Multifocal concentric luminal narrowing alternates with areas of mural dilatation ("string of beads").
- *Intracranial atherosclerosis:* Although the angiographic findings may be similar, multiple intracranial stenoses in a young patient are unlikely to be the result of atherosclerosis.

### ■ Essential Facts

- Central nervous system vasculitis is a cause of stroke in young people.
- It may present with intracerebral or subarachnoid hemorrhage.
- Multiple infarcts of various ages are present in more than one vascular territory.
- Large-vessel vasculitis affects the ICA, the M1 and A1 segments, the intracranial vertebral artery, the basilar artery, and the P1 segment. It may present after varicella-zoster virus infection or bacterial meningitis.
- Medium-vessel vasculitis occurs in panarteritis nodosa, lupus erythematosus, Behçet disease, Crohn disease, and Sneddon syndrome.
- Small-vessel vasculitis occurs in leukocytoclastic vasculitis.

### ■ Other Imaging Findings

- Angiography reveals one or multiple stenoses of brain vessels and abnormal straightening and kinking of arteries caused by vessel wall induration and multiple microaneurysms.
- Contrast enhancement of the vessel wall has been described.
- Conventional angiography is the gold standard.
- Brain biopsy may be necessary for the diagnosis.
- High-resolution magnetic resonance (MR) imaging of the skull base with contrast enhancement may demonstrate vessel wall thickening.

### ✓ Pearls & ✗ Pitfalls

- ✓ MR angiography (MRA) may demonstrate irregularity of the intracranial vessels in the three-dimensional reconstructions when there is motion artifact. Careful review of the source images helps to determine if the MRA is of diagnostic quality.
- ✗ Intracranial MRA may suggest complete occlusion of vessels with severe stenosis and decreased flow.

# Case 60

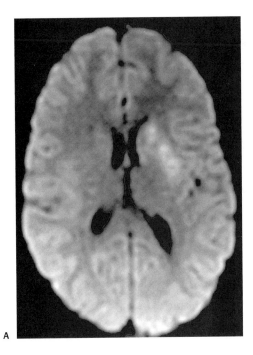

A

## Clinical Presentation

A 17-year-old girl who fainted while playing basketball.

## Further Work-up

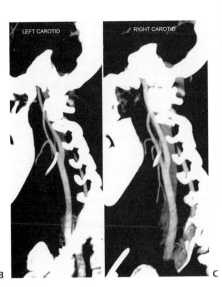

B

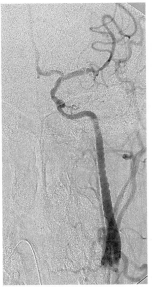

C

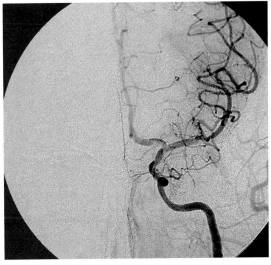

D

## ■ Imaging Findings

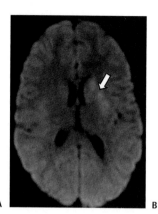
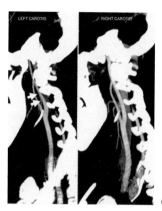
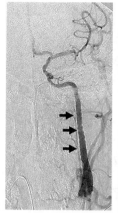
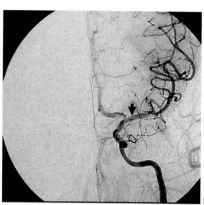

**(A)** Diffusion-weighted image demonstrates acute ischemic changes in the left caudate head and putamen (*arrow*). **(B)** Sagittal computed tomography angiography maximum-intensity-projection images of the bifurcations of both carotid arteries demonstrate long-segment narrowing of the left internal carotid artery (ICA) with a serrated contour (*arrows*). **(C)** Lateral projection of a digital subtraction angiogram of the left ICA shows a "string of beads" appearance in the cervical segment (*arrows*). **(D)** Intracranial views of the same injection show a linear filling defect in the proximal left middle cerebral artery, consistent with a dissection flap (*arrow*). Irregular filling defects in the distal carotid artery and anterior cerebral artery are also noted, which represent thrombi.

## ■ Differential Diagnosis

- **Fibromuscular dysplasia (FMD):** FMD is an infrequent cause of stroke in young people. It is characterized by a multifocal concentric luminal narrowing alternating with areas of mural dilatation that are wider than the original lumen. It may be associated with arterial dissection.
- *Atherosclerotic narrowing:* This frequently involves the carotid bifurcation and carotid siphons. Long-segment stenosis is infrequent. It is not usually seen in young patients.
- *Mechanically induced vasospasm:* This is a mechanically induced contraction of smooth-muscle fibers in the wall of a vessel. It is a common adverse event that may complicate an endovascular procedure by limiting distal blood flow. It has a "standing waves" appearance that mimics FMD. This is a transient phenomenon that usually resolves after withdrawal of the offending catheter.

## ■ Essential Facts

- FMD is a nonatherosclerotic, noninflammatory arterial disease that most commonly involves the renal and carotid arteries.
- Cervicocranial FMD is often asymptomatic and can manifest with transient ischemic attack, amaurosis fugax, stroke, or nonspecific symptoms such as headache and tinnitus.
- FMD may be associated with arterial dissection, intracranial aneurysms, and arteriovenous fistulas.

## ■ Other Imaging Findings

- Angiography reveals multifocal concentric luminal narrowing alternating with areas of mural dilatation that are wider than the original lumen ("string of beads"), focal or tubular stenosis, a septum, or a diverticulum.
- Computed tomography angiography and magnetic resonance angiography (MRA) are effective for detecting lesions of the middle and distal portions of the carotid and vertebral arteries and may also document or rule out the association of intracranial aneurysms.

## ✓ Pearls & ✗ Pitfalls

- ✓ Unlike atherosclerotic stenoses, stenoses arising from FMD rarely affect the ostial or proximal segments of arteries.
- ✓ Spontaneous cervical artery dissections are a common cause of stroke in young and middle-aged adults and are associated with FMD in ~15% of cases.
- ✗ On time-of-flight MRA, artifacts caused by patient motion and swallowing or related to in-plane flow and susceptibility gradients may mimic the appearance of FMD and tend to decrease both the sensitivity and specificity of this modality for the detection of cervicocephalic FMD.

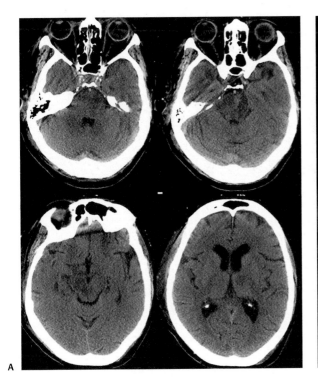
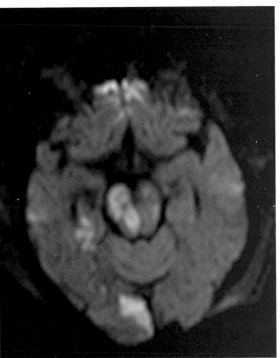

# Case 61

A

B

## Clinical Presentation

A 70-year-old woman presenting with syncope after a fall.

**Further Work-up**

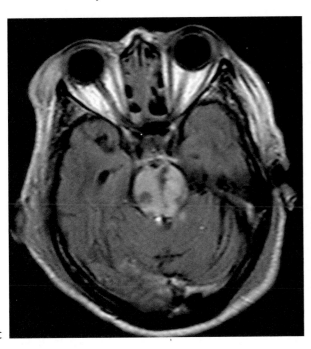

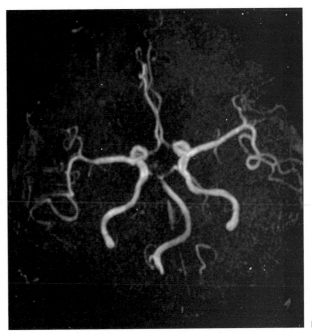

C

D

### ■ Imaging Findings

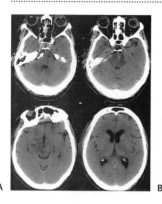 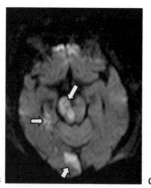 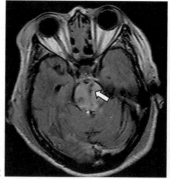 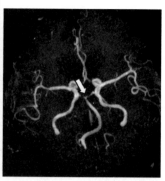

**(A)** Computed tomography (CT) of the brain shows areas of low attenuation in the pons, right cerebral peduncle, and left thalamus. Note the increased attenuation of the basilar artery (*arrow*). **(B)** Diffusion-weighted image shows restricted diffusion in the right side of the pons, right medial temporal lobe, and right occipital lobe (*arrows*). All the areas of hypoattenuation on the CT scan demonstrate restriction (not all of them shown). **(C)** Fluid-attenuated inversion recovery image through the pons shows increased signal and punctate areas of hemorrhage (*arrow*). **(D)** Magnetic resonance angiography (MRA) of the brain shows no flow-related signal in the basilar tip or proximal posterior cerebral arteries (*arrow*). The superior cerebellar arteries are irregular and narrow.

### ■ Differential Diagnosis

- *Basilar artery thrombosis with acute posterior circulation stroke:* Acute ischemic changes involve variable extensions of the brainstem, cerebellum, thalami, and temporal and occipital lobes. Edema in the posterior fossa may result in obliteration of the 4th ventricle and acute hydrocephalus.
- *Osmotic demyelination, also known as central pontine myelinolysis (CPM):* Osmotic demyelination is a localized, frequently symmetric, noninflammatory demyelination within the central pons. In 10% of patients, demyelination is present in extrapontine regions, including the midbrain, thalami, basal nuclei, and cerebellum. CPM occurs inconsistently as a complication of severe and prolonged hyponatremia, particularly when it is corrected too rapidly. T2-weighted magnetic resonance imaging (MRI) shows hyperintense areas where demyelination has occurred.
- *Thrombosis of the deep cerebral veins:* This causes symmetric infarcts that affect the thalami bilaterally, possibly extending into the basal ganglia and adjacent white matter bilaterally. The venous structures, such as the thalamostriate vein, internal carotid vein, vein of Rosenthal, vein of Galen, straight sinus, and torcular, are hyperattenuated on CT. Hydrocephalus may occur as a consequence of edema and swelling of both thalami.

### ■ Essential Facts

- Variable symptoms result from ischemia of the cerebellum, brainstem, occipital lobes, and thalami.
- Vascular territories:
  - The posterior inferior cerebellar artery (PICA) and the anterior inferior cerebellar artery supply the inferior cerebellum and lateral aspects of the medulla and pons, respectively.

- The superior cerebellar artery supplies the superior cerebellum, including the superior cerebellar peduncle, as well as the upper dorsolateral pons and midbrain.
- Basilar artery branches (perforators) supply the paramedian and anterolateral brainstem.
- The proximal posterior cerebral artery, referred to as the precommunicating or P1 segment, supplies regions of the midbrain, mammillary body, and optic tract.
- Mechanism of basilar artery occlusion:
  - Most cases of distal (top of the basilar artery) or proximal (vertebrobasilar junction) occlusion are caused by embolism from either a cardiac or an arterial source.
  - Midbasilar artery occlusion is typically the result of atherothrombosis.
  - Arterial dissections are very rare and usually involve the vertebral artery, with occasional extension to the basilar artery.

### ■ Other Imaging Findings

- The sensitivity of CT to detect posterior circulation stroke is poor.
- MRI and MRA are highly sensitive to detect acute ischemia and arterial occlusion.
- MRA may overestimate the degree of stenosis because of reduced flow.

### ✓ Pearls & ✗ Pitfalls

- ✓ Top-of-the-basilar syndrome: severe impairment of consciousness, usually bilateral oculomotor palsies, visual fields defects, cerebellar symptoms, and hemiplegia or tetraplegia
- ✓ Results from thalamic, occipital, and cerebellar infarctions
- ✗ A hypoplastic vertebral artery may terminate in the PICA without connecting to the basilar artery. This finding can be mistaken for occlusion.

# Case 62

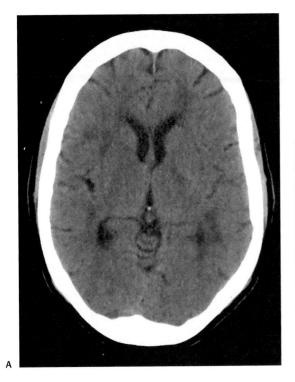

A

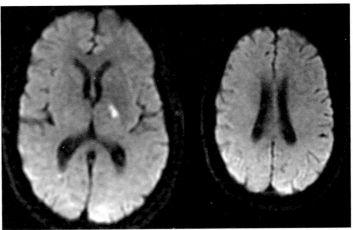

B

## Clinical Presentation

A 47-year-old woman with transient weakness.

## Further Work-up

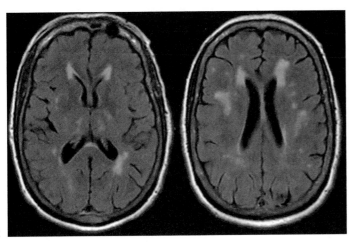

C

## ■ Imaging Findings

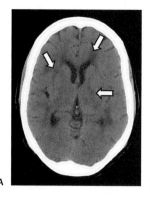
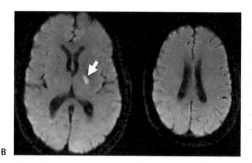
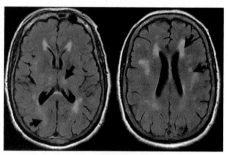

**(A)** Computed tomography (CT) of the brain shows numerous small areas of low attenuation in the deep white matter bilaterally and in the left thalamus (*arrows*). **(B)** Diffusion-weighted image shows restriction in the left thalamus (*arrow*). The centrum semiovale is unremarkable. **(C)** Fluid-attenuated inversion recovery (FLAIR) images demonstrate numerous areas of high signal (*arrows*), including the lesion with restricted diffusion in the left thalamus.

## ■ Differential Diagnosis

- ***Acute and chronic lacunar infarcts:*** These present as multiple small areas of T2 signal abnormality; if magnetic resonance imaging (MRI) is acquired in the acute phase, there is restricted diffusion. The distribution is not typical for demyelinating lesions.
- *Multiple sclerosis (MS):* MS is an inflammatory, demyelinating disease of the central nervous system. On MRI, typical MS appears as oval areas of T2 hyperintensity in the periventricular regions, with their longest axis oriented perpendicular to the ventricular surface. White matter lesions involving the corpus callosum, infratentorial compartment, and spinal cord make the diagnosis of MS more likely. Enhancement and restricted diffusion are seen in active lesions.
- *Migraine-related ischemic lesions:* There is an increased frequency of small white matter lesions in patients with a history of migraine headaches. These are believed to represent subclinical infarcts.

## ■ Essential Facts

- Lacunes are small subcortical infarcts (< 15 mm in diameter) in the territory of the deep penetrating arteries.
- Lacunar infarcts may be asymptomatic, or patients may present with specific lacunar syndromes: pure motor stroke/hemiparesis, ataxic hemiparesis, dysarthria/clumsy hand, pure sensory stroke, or mixed sensorimotor stroke
- They occur most frequently in the basal ganglia and internal capsule, thalamus, corona radiata, and pons.
- Associated conditions include hypertension, smoking, diabetes, and microemboli from the heart or carotid arteries.

## ■ Other Imaging Findings

- CT findings may be normal, or a small area of low attenuation may be seen. The age of lacunar infarcts is difficult to establish with CT.
- MRI demonstrates restricted diffusion. A few hours later, a T2 signal increase is also present.

## ✓ Pearls & ✗ Pitfalls

- ✓ Other forms of arteriopathy that can affect small vessels include amyloid angiopathy, hemodynamic disorders, and cerebral autosomal-dominant arteriopathy with subcortical infarcts and leukoencephalopathy (CADASIL).
- ✓ Abnormalities in the perfusion studies may predict progression of a lacunar stroke.
- ✗ Virchow-Robin spaces are extensions of the subarachnoid space surrounding the blood vessels and should not be mistaken for lacunar infarcts. They follow the signal of cerebrospinal fluid on all sequences. Increased FLAIR signal or restricted diffusion should not be present.

# Case 63

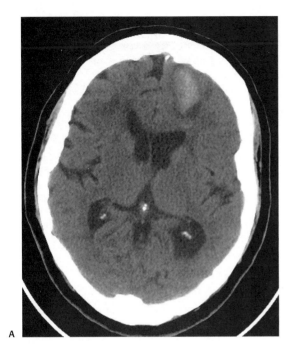

A

## ■ Clinical Presentation

A 78-year-old man with a history of prior cerebral hemorrhage presenting with headache and right leg weakness.

## Further Work-up

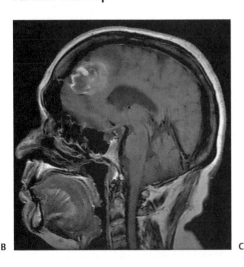

B

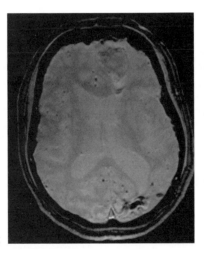

C

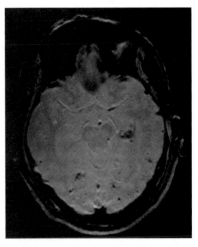

D

### ■ Imaging Findings

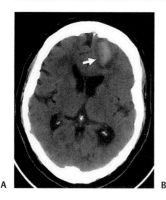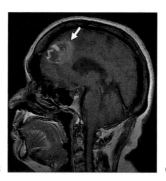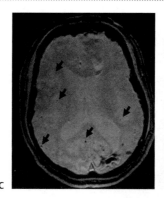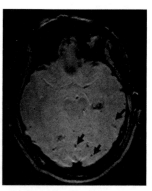

A    B    C    D

**(A)** Nonenhanced computed tomography (CT) of the brain demonstrates acute hemorrhage in the left frontal lobe (*arrow*). **(B)** Sagittal T1-weighted image (WI) of the brain shows a subacute hematoma in the right frontal lobe (*arrow*). **(C)** Gradient-echo (GRE) T2*WI shows an acute left frontal hematoma, an old left occipital hemorrhagic lesion, and multiple punctate foci of hemosiderin deposition in the subcortical regions of both cerebral hemispheres (*arrows*). **(D)** GRE T2*WI: note the multiple punctate foci of hemosiderin deposition in both cerebral hemispheres (*arrows*).

### ■ Differential Diagnosis

- ***Intracranial hemorrhage (ICH) secondary to cerebral amyloid angiopathy (CAA):*** CAA causes multiple and recurrent ICH in a cortical-subcortical distribution that generally spares the deep white matter, basal ganglia, and brainstem. It may involve the cerebellum. Subarachnoid and subdural hemorrhage (may be primary or due to direct extension of the cortical-subcortical hemorrhage) can also occur. Cortical microhemorrhages can be better visualized on GRE T2*-weighted magnetic resonance imaging (MRI).
- *Hypertensive ICH:* Hypertension is the most common cause of nontraumatic hemorrhage in adults. In contrast to the typical cortical-subcortical location of CAA-related hemorrhage, hypertensive hemorrhages, both large and small, most commonly occur in the deep gray matter, such as the basal ganglia and thalami, or in the brainstem.
- *Hemorrhagic metastasis:* The intracerebral metastases most prone to hemorrhage include malignant melanoma, choriocarcinoma, renal cell carcinoma, bronchogenic carcinoma, and thyroid malignancy. Of the primary gliomas, glioblastoma multiforme, oligodendroglioma, and ependymoma are the ones that can present with hemorrhage.

### ■ Essential Facts

- CAA is an important cause of spontaneous cortical-subcortical ICH in the normotensive elderly.
- There may be deposition of β-amyloid protein in the media and adventitia of small and medium-size vessels of the cerebral cortex, subcortex, and leptomeninges.
- The clinical presentation includes sudden neurologic deficit (stroke) related to acute ICH and symptoms resembling those of a transient ischemic attack or dementia.

### ■ Other Imaging Findings

- CT shows acute hemorrhage or encephalomalacia from prior bleeding. Leukoaraiosis is frequently present.
- GRE T2*-weighted MRI is used to evaluate for microhemorrhages.

### ✓ Pearls & ✗ Pitfalls

- ✓ Cerebral microhemorrhages can be seen in patients with CAA and chronic systemic hypertension most commonly.
- ✓ Other causes of ICH include diffuse axonal injury, cerebral embolism, cerebral autosomal-dominant arteriopathy with subcortical infarcts and leukoencephalopathy (CADASIL), multiple cavernous malformations, vasculitis, hemorrhagic micrometastasis, and radiation vasculopathy.
- ✗ Increased T1 signal intensity in a hematoma should not be mistaken for enhancement.

# Case 64

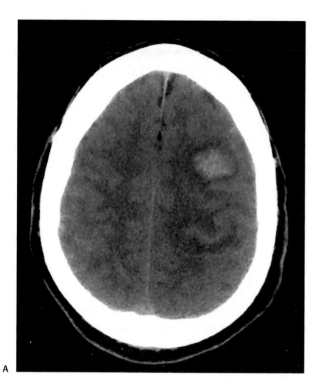

A

## Clinical Presentation

A 72-year-old man with a history of treated cancer, now presenting with severe headache.

## Further Work-up

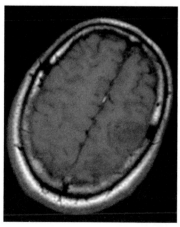

B

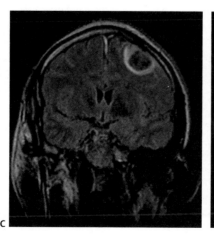

C

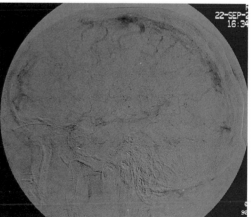

D

## ■ Imaging Findings

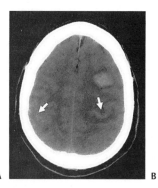
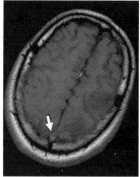
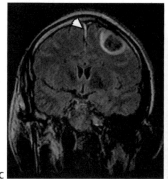
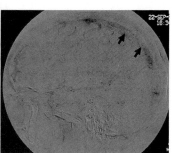

A    B    C    D

**(A)** Axial computed tomography (CT) of the brain demonstrates subarachnoid hemorrhage at the vertex bilaterally (*arrows*) and parenchymal hematoma in the left frontal lobe. **(B)** Axial T1-weighted image (WI) shows increased signal in the superior longitudinal sinus (*arrow*). The left frontal hematoma is isointense to the cortex (acute). **(C)** Coronal T2WI shows subdural hemorrhage in the parafalcine region (*arrowhead*). The parenchymal hematoma shows a central area of low signal and a rim of high signal. **(D)** Lateral projection digital subtraction angiography of the venous phase of the left carotid injection demonstrates multiple filling defects in the sagittal sinus (*arrows*).

## ■ Differential Diagnosis

- ***Parenchymal and extra-axial hemorrhages secondary to venous sinus thrombosis:*** Parenchymal hemorrhage can be seen in one-third of cases of cerebral venous thrombosis. Hemorrhages are typically cortical with subcortical extension. Smaller zones of isolated subcortical hemorrhage also may be seen.
- *Bleeding metastasis:* This may be single or multiple, and simultaneous extra-axial hemorrhage is usually absent. Additional nonhemorrhagic metastatic lesions with mass effect and vasogenic edema are frequently seen.
- *Dural arteriovenous fistula:* The clinical presentation may be identical to that of sinus thrombosis. Increased venous pressure may result in thrombosis. Conventional angiography demonstrates the arteriovenous shunt in the dura.

## ■ Essential Facts

- The clinical presentation includes headache, focal neurologic deficits, and seizures.
- Parenchymal changes include infarctions in a nonarterial distribution in the white matter and/or cortical–white matter junction and early hemorrhagic transformation.
- Flame-shaped irregular zones of lobar hemorrhage in the parasagittal frontal and parietal lobes are typical findings in patients with superior sagittal sinus thrombosis.
- Treatment options are anticoagulation with heparin and endovascular recanalization.

## ■ Other Imaging Findings

- Signs of sinus occlusion are the following: delta sign on noncontrast-enhanced CT (dense triangle from hyperdense thrombus within the sinus), reverse delta sign on contrast-enhanced CT (empty triangle from enhancement of the dural leaves surrounding the comparatively less dense thrombosed sinus).
- Magnetic resonance (MR) imaging: the signal intensity of the thrombus varies with time.
- Time-of-flight (TOF) MR venography is the method most commonly used for the diagnosis of cerebral venous thrombosis. Two planes of acquisition improve the assessment of all the sinuses.
- Contrast-enhanced MR venography is better than TOF MR venography to visualize small vessels.
- CT venography provides a highly detailed depiction of the cerebral venous system, superior to that available with conventional TOF MR venography, and has at least equivalent accuracy for the detection of cerebral venous thrombosis.

## ✓ Pearls & ✗ Pitfalls

- ✓ Restricted diffusion may or may not be seen in cerebral venous thrombosis; when present, it may be reversible.
- ✗ An intrasinus thrombus in the subacute stage may have markedly increased signal intensity on MR images that may be misinterpreted as evidence of flow on TOF MR venograms. A close evaluation of MR venographic source images usually allows differentiation, as the thrombus signal is typically not as intense as the flow-related signal.

# Case 65

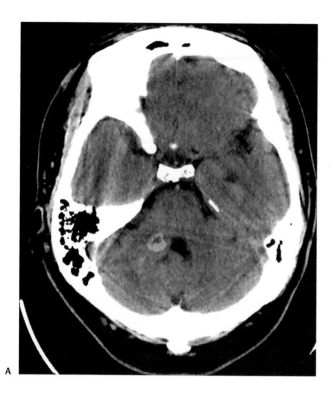

A

## Clinical Presentation

A 35-year-old with the new onset of seizures.

## Further Work-up

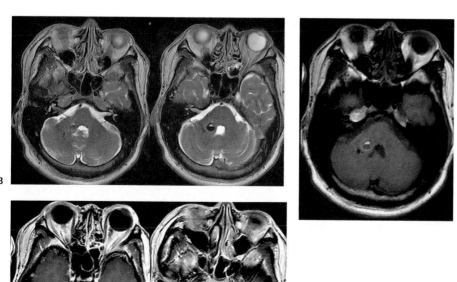

B

C

D

### ■ Imaging Findings

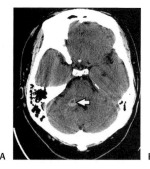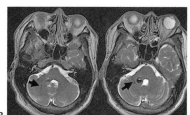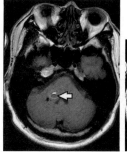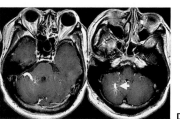

A  B  C  D

**(A)** Nonenhanced computed tomography (CT) demonstrates a round area of increased attenuation with a fluidlike core in the right middle cerebellar peduncle (*arrow*). There is no edema or mass effect. **(B)** Axial T2-weighted images (WIs) show a round lesion with heterogeneous intensity. A rim of low signal is evident. There are a few linear flow voids lateral to this lesion (*arrows*). **(C)** The areas of high signal on T2WIs are also hyperintense on T1WIs. The dark rim on T2WIs has intermediate signal on T1WIs. Findings are consistent with blood products of different ages (*arrow*). **(D)** Axial T1WIs after contrast show enhancement of vascular structures, with a linear and a "caput medusae" pattern (*arrow*).

### ■ Differential Diagnosis

- ***Cavernous malformation (CM) with associated developmental venous anomaly (DVA):*** CMs are vascular malformations composed of well-circumscribed sinusoidal vascular channels containing blood in various stages of evolution. The lesion is well defined and lobulated, with a reticulated core of heterogeneous T1 and T2 signal as a result of thrombosis, fibrosis, calcification, and hemorrhage. Associated DVA shows a flow void in the draining vein.
- *Arteriovenous malformation:* This causes variable hemorrhage and gliosis of the adjacent parenchyma and enlargement of the feeding arteries and draining veins. A nidus may be identified on the T2WI, postcontrast T1WI, or conventional angiogram.
- *Hemangioblastoma:* This is the most common primary intra-axial posterior fossa tumor in adults. The second most common location is the spinal cord. Twenty-five percent of all cases are associated with von Hippel-Lindau disease. CT and magnetic resonance imaging (MRI) typically show an enhancing tumor nodule in association with an adjacent cyst.
- CMs are also known as cavernomas, cavernous angiomas,

### ■ Essential Facts

angiographically occult vascular malformations, or cavernous hemangiomas.
- CMs may be asymptomatic, or they may present clinically with headache, seizures, and hemorrhage.
- CMs may be congenital or arise de novo in familial cases and after radiation, pregnancy, or brain biopsy.
- CMs are associated with DVAs (congenital variants of cerebral venous drainage without involvement of capillaries or arteries).

### ■ Other Imaging Findings

- On CT, there is increased attenuation (from calcium, blood, or both) with indistinct margins, a stippled appearance, and no mass effect.
- On T2WIs, a signal void is seen in the draining vein; variable degrees of T2 and T1 prolongation may be present in the adjacent parenchyma.
- Contrast-enhanced MRI may show the associated DVA as a series of small, deep parenchymal veins converging toward a larger collecting vein, which follows a transhemispheric course before draining into a normal deep or superficial vein.
- There is a rim of low signal on gradient-echo and T2WIs from hemosiderin and iron deposition in the adjacent parenchyma.
- At angiography, a DVA typically opacifies at the same time as the normal veins, although DVAs in the frontal lobes may opacify earlier with an associated capillary blush.

### ✔ Pearls & ✘ Pitfalls

- ✔ Magnetic resonance perfusion of DVAs can show an association with varying degrees of elevation in the cerebral blood volume, mean transit time, and time to peak.
- ✘ Recent hemorrhage in a cavernous anomaly may result in an atypical appearance, with perilesional and extralesional hemorrhage outside the hemosiderin ring, an increase in size with respect to prior studies, edema, or mass effect.
- ✘ Follow-up imaging is warranted in these cases.

# Case 66

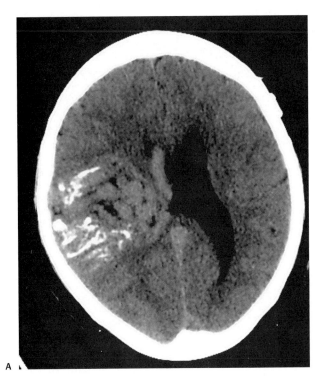

A

## Clinical Presentation

A 55-year-old woman with headaches and left hemiparesis.

## Further Work-up

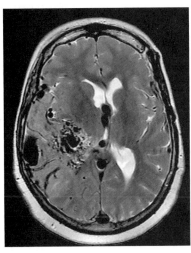

B

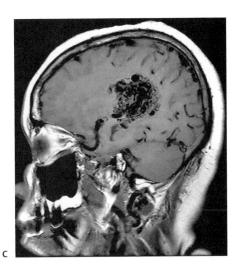

C

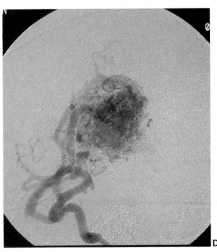

D

■ **Imaging Findings**

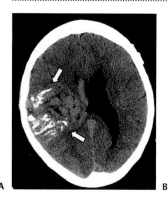
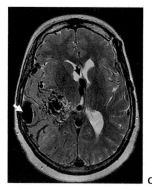
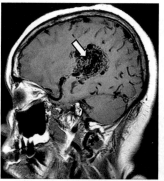
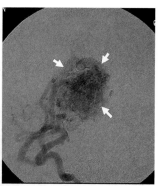

A B C D

**(A)** Computed tomography (CT) of the brain shows a large right hemispheric lesion with linear calcifications and serpentine areas of increased attenuation (*arrows*). Note that the mass effect of the lesion is small relative to its size. **(B)** Axial T2-weighted image (WI) shows numerous large flow voids surrounded by areas of high signal in the temporal and parietal lobes, indicative of gliosis. The internal cerebral veins (*black arrow*) and superficial veins (*white arrow*) are enlarged. **(C)** Sagittal T1WI shows flow voids in a large arteriovenous nidus (*arrow*). **(D)** Right internal carotid angiogram shows early filling of a large arteriovenous nidus (*arrows*).

■ **Differential Diagnosis**

- *Arteriovenous malformation (AVM):* AVM is a vascular malformation in which blood flows directly from the arterial system to the venous system without passing through a capillary system (i.e., arteriovenous shunt). Calcifications occur in 25 to 30% of cases. There is strong serpentine enhancement. Magnetic resonance (MR) imaging demonstrates tightly packed flow voids, high T2 signal due to gliosis, and enlarged arterial feeders or draining veins. Blood products of various ages are seen.
- *Highly vascular glioma:* This presents as an enhancing mass in which prominent intratumoral vessels are the predominant feature. There is significant mass effect and surrounding edema. Angiogram shows tumor blush without enlarged draining veins.
- *Sturge-Weber syndrome:* This is also called *encephalotrigeminal angiomatosis.* It is a neurocutaneous disorder in which angiomas involve the leptomeninges and skin of the face. The abnormal venous drainage of the hemispheres results in the enlargement of collateral veins from the choroid plexus and medullary veins. Chronic cerebral ischemia leads to atrophy and calcification (described as a "tram track" appearance).

■ **Essential Facts**

- AVMs are lesions of the cerebral vasculature.
- The clinical presentation includes hemorrhage, seizure, headache, and progressive neurologic deficit. In pediatric patients, there may also be heart failure, macrocephaly, and prominent scalp veins.
- AVMs have enlarged feeding arteries and draining veins and an arteriovenous nidus.
- Gliosis in the adjacent brain parenchyma is associated with evidence of recent or remote hemorrhage.
- Treatment consists of surgery, stereotactic radiosurgery, and embolization, alone or in combination.

■ **Other Imaging Findings**

- On CT, an AVM appears as an iso- or hyperattenuating mass with limited mass effect relative to its size.
- CT angiography and MR angiography are helpful to delineate the architecture of the lesion, demonstrate and measure the nidus, and plan treatment; however, they lack the dynamic information that conventional angiography provides.
- Conventional cerebral angiography is the gold standard for characterizing the lesion and planning treatment.

✓ **Pearls & ✗ Pitfalls**

- ✓ The Spetzler-Martin grading system helps predict the likelihood of a satisfactory outcome if surgical resection is attempted.
- ✓ Grades are assigned depending on the size of the nidus, eloquence of the adjacent brain parenchyma, and deep versus superficial venous drainage.
- ✓ Eloquent areas include the sensorimotor, language, and visual cortex; thalami; hypothalamus; internal capsules; brainstem; cerebellar peduncles, and deep cerebellar nuclei.
- ✗ Thrombi within an AVM may simulate hemorrhage.

# Case 67

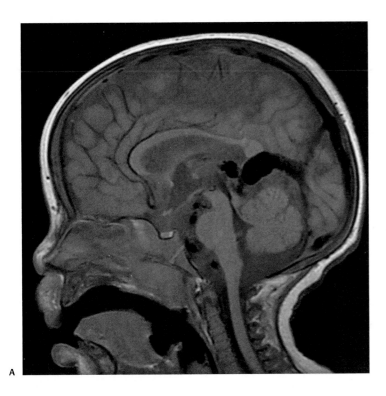

A

## Clinical Presentation

A premature infant with cardiac failure.

## Further Work-up

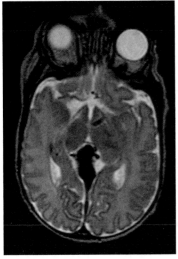

B

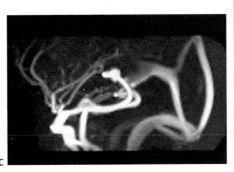

C

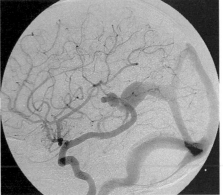

D

## Imaging Findings

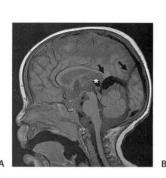
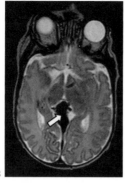
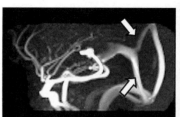
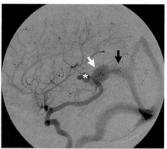

A  B  C  D

**(A)** Sagittal T1-weighted image (WI) shows large flow voids in the region of the tectum (*asterisk*) and prominent midline veins in the margin of the tentorium and occipital region (*arrows*). **(B)** Axial T2WI confirms prominent veins in the tectal region (*arrow*). **(C)** Sagittal phase-contrast magnetic resonance (MR) venogram shows enlarged veins from the tectum to the torcula and sagittal sinus (*arrows*). **(D)** Digital subtracted angiogram of a left internal carotid injection shows a prominent posterior communicating artery and posterior cerebral artery shunting into a venous pouch (*asterisk*) located anterosuperiorly to the dilated vein of Galen (*white arrow*), which subsequently drains into a falcine sinus (*black arrow*) toward the sagittal sinus and torcula.

## Differential Diagnosis

- *Vein of Galen aneurysmal malformation (VGAM):* VGAM is characterized by prominent arteries and veins in the tectum that converge toward a dilated vein of Galen. It is a frequent cause of heart failure in neonates and can be diagnosed in utero.
- *Thrombosis of the torcular Herophili:* Venous obstructions would result in venous infarcts and hemorrhages, as well as enlarged collateral veins. A lack of flow would be evident in the obstructed sinus.

## Essential Facts

- VGAMs are rare congenital vascular malformations characterized by the shunting of arterial flow into an enlarged cerebral vein dorsal to the tectum.
- VGAMs are thought to result from the development of an arteriovenous connection between primitive choroidal vessels and the median prosencephalic vein of Markowski.
- The abnormal flow through the connection retards the normal involution of this embryonic vein and thus prevents the development of the vein of Galen.
- Clinical presentation:
  - High-output heart failure in the newborn
  - Strokes or steal phenomena
  - Hemorrhage (uncommon)
  - Hydrocephalus
- Treatment is endovascular embolization.
- MR angiography can help to delineate the vascular supply.
- Venous anatomy is well shown by MR venography.

## Other Imaging Findings

- Ultrasound can demonstrate the malformation in the fetal period.
- Computed tomography angiography simultaneously depicts the venous and arterial anatomy. The use of iodinated contrast material should be limited in children with a shunt because of the risk for renal dysfunction.
- Cerebral angiography defines the extent of aneurysmal dilatation and details the arterial supply.

## ✓ Pearls & ✗ Pitfalls

- ✓ Lasjaunias and colleagues have separated VGAMs from vein of Galen aneurysmal dilatations (VGADs).
- ✓ In VGADs, a parenchymal arteriovenous malformation drains through the vein of Galen. The dilated vein in these cases drains both brain parenchyma and the malformation, whereas the persistent embryonic vein in the true VGAM drains only the malformation.
- ✓ Patients with VGADs more often present with intracranial hemorrhage.
- ✗ The VGAM may result in hydrocephalus. However, shunting before obliteration of the VGAM is usually avoided because it has been reported to worsen cerebral perfusion.

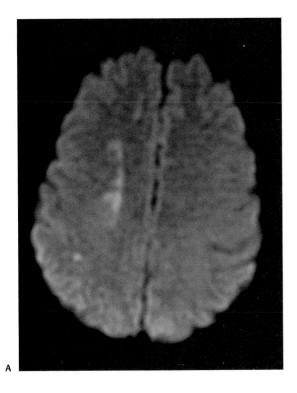

# Case 68

A

## Clinical Presentation

A 75-year-old woman presenting with transient left hemiparesis.

## Further Work-up

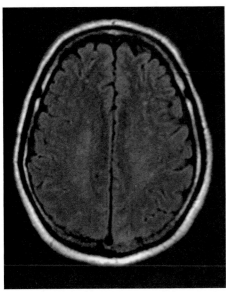

B

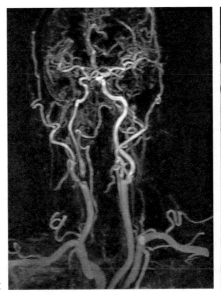

C

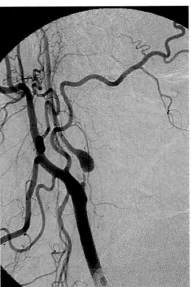

D

■ **Imaging Findings**

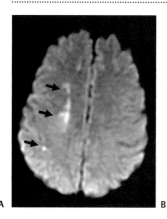 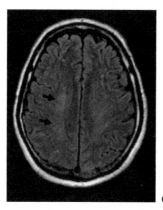 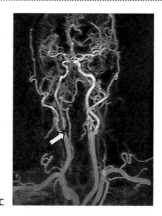 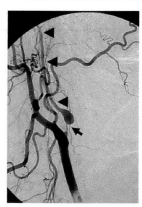

A    B    C    D

**(A)** Diffusion image demonstrates ischemic changes in the so-called internal watershed in the deep white matter between the territories of the anterior cerebral artery and middle cerebral artery on the right (*arrows*). **(B)** Very subtle T2 signal changes are present in the same area on the fluid-attenuated inversion recovery image (*arrows*). **(C)** Magnetic resonance angiography (MRA) of the neck with contrast demonstrates signal dropout in the proximal right internal carotid artery (ICA), which is consistent with critical stenosis (*arrow*). The degree of stenosis cannot be quantified. **(D)** Critical stenosis (>90%) in the proximal ICA is confirmed on the digital subtraction angiogram (DSA; *arrow*). The diameter of the distal ICA (*arrowheads*) is small compared with that of the contralateral ICA (not shown).

■ **Differential Diagnosis**

- **Critical ICA stenosis:** Infarcts in the watershed territories may result solely from hemodynamic compromise, but they are more frequent in the setting of carotid stenosis.
- *Carotid pseudoaneurysm:* Traumatic disruption of the continuity of the arterial wall results in periarterial hematoma contained by adjacent soft tissues. Subsequent encapsulation results in pseudoaneurysm formation. Other signs of vascular trauma, such as stenosis, dissection, and occlusion, may be present.
- *Carotid dissection:* This more frequently manifests as a long segment of smooth luminal narrowing. False and true lumina may be demonstrated. Carotid dissection is associated with pseudoaneurysm.

■ **Essential Facts**

- Atherosclerotic disease of the cervical carotid artery is a frequent cause of stroke.
- Infarcts may occur in the cortical watershed or in the internal watershed (rosary-like pattern in the centrum semiovale).
- Mechanism of stroke:
  - Thromboembolism develops from atherosclerotic plaque.
  - Low-flow states affect the territory of penetrating arterioles from the most distal middle and anterior cerebral arteries, which have no potential for collateral supply.
  - Most strokes likely represent a synergistic effect of the two mechanisms.
- Indications for imaging of the carotid arteries are carotid bruit, transient ischemic attack, and ischemic stroke.
- According to the North American Symptomatic Carotid Endarterectomy Trial (NASCET), symptomatic and asymp-

tomatic patients with carotid stenosis of at least 70% will benefit from carotid endarterectomy.
- When the residual luminal diameter is less than 1 mm, the carotid artery distal to the stenosis narrows because of a decrease in the perfusion pressure.

■ **Other Imaging Findings**

- Conventional angiography is the gold standard for the quantification of stenosis.
- Two noninvasive methods, such as ultrasound, computed tomography angiography (CTA), or MRA, can be used instead of conventional angiography, provided that the findings are concordant.
- The quantification of the degree of stenosis by conventional angiography, CTA, and MRA is based on NASCET criteria for comparing the diameter of the residual lumen to that of the distal ICA.
- In duplex ultrasound, the degree of stenosis is estimated based on the correlation of velocity measurements with angiographic stenosis.

✓ **Pearls & ✗ Pitfalls**

✓ Carotid duplex imaging can be limited by the presence of dense calcifications in the carotid plaque.
✓ In MRA, flow-related signal dropout occurs in areas of turbulent or vortex flow.
✓ Metallic stents cause signal dropout that limits MRA interpretation.
✓ The assessment of stenosis by CTA can be limited by heavily calcified or circumferential plaques.
✗ In DSA or CTA, the ascending pharyngeal artery can be mistaken for a hairline ICA in cases of carotid occlusion.

# Case 69

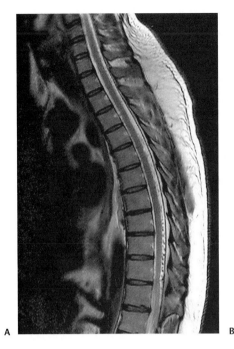
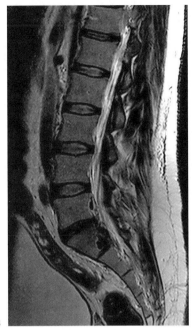
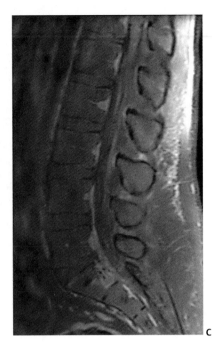

A

B

C

## ■ Clinical Presentation

A 38-year-old man with lower extremity numbness and progressive weakness.

## Further Work-up

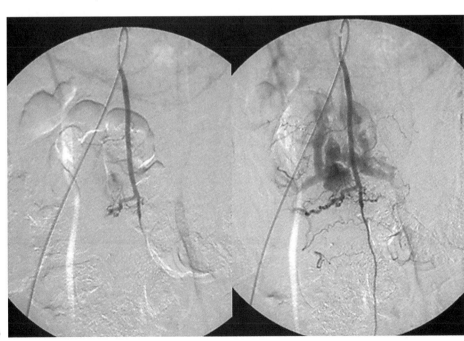

D

### ■ Imaging Findings

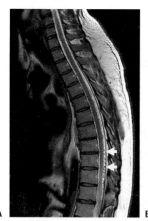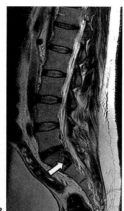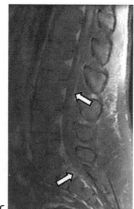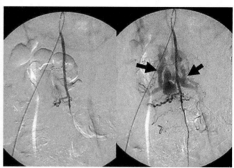

**(A)** Sagittal T2–weighted image (WI) of the thoracic spine shows multiple tiny flow voids in the posterior subarachnoid space (*arrows*). **(B)** Sagittal T2WI of the lumbar spine shows a tangle of vessels causing scalloping of the posterior margin of the S1 vertebral body (*arrow*). **(C)** Sagittal postcontrast T1WI in the lumbar region shows enhancement of the vascular structures within the thecal sac and epidural space (*arrows*). **(D)** Lateral projection of a spinal angiogram with injection in the artery of Adamkiewicz shows early opacification of large veins (*arrows*) in the epidural and subarachnoid spaces. No nidus is identified.

### ■ Differential Diagnosis

- **Spinal dural arteriovenous fistula:** The fistula causes vessel dilatation and tortuosity, evidenced by signal voids around the cord. Gadolinium enhancement often facilitates recognition of the vessels. There may be T2 signal abnormality and patchy enhancement of the involved cord.
- *Arachnoiditis:* Arachnoiditis is inflammation of the meninges and subarachnoid space secondary to infectious, inflammatory, or neoplastic processes. T2WIs show loculation and obliteration of the subarachnoid space. The nerve roots show irregularity, clumping, and thickening. Peripheral adherence of the nerve roots to the walls of the thecal sac produces the so-called featureless, or empty, sac. There may be enhancement.
- *Leptomeningeal carcinomatosis:* Diffuse seeding of the leptomeninges by tumor metastases occurs most commonly in adults with breast carcinoma, lung carcinoma, or melanoma and in children with hematogenous malignancies or primitive neuroectodermal tumor. On magnetic resonance (MR) imaging, there is peripheral linear or nodular enhancement of the pia mater. In addition, enhancement of the nerve roots within the cauda equina is often seen, ranging from tiny nodules to large masses.

### ■ Essential Facts

- Spinal vascular malformations comprise dural arteriovenous fistulas (DAVFs) and arteriovenous malformations (AVMs).
  - DAVFs: acquired; fed by radiculomeningeal arteries; shunt located in the dura, near the spinal nerve root; venous congestion and intramedullary edema leading to chronic hypoxic myelopathy; treated with surgical ligation of the vein or glue embolization

- AVMs: inborn; fed by radiculomedullary (cord) arteries; intra- or perimedullary shunt; may have a nidus or a fistulous transition from artery to vein; venous congestion, hemorrhage, steal phenomenon
- Selective spinal angiography is necessary to define the type of malformation and plan treatment.

### ✓ Pearls & ✗ Pitfalls

- ✓ A complete spinal angiogram includes selective injections of the intercostal, lumbar, and internal iliac arteries. If no fistula is found, then the blood supply to the cervical spine, as well as the intracranial circulation, should be studied.
- ✓ Contrast-enhanced MR angiography may help to localize the enlarged feeders before conventional angiography.
- ✗ Small vascular flow voids are usually present within the spinal subarachnoid space without mass effect or cord signal abnormality.

# Case 70

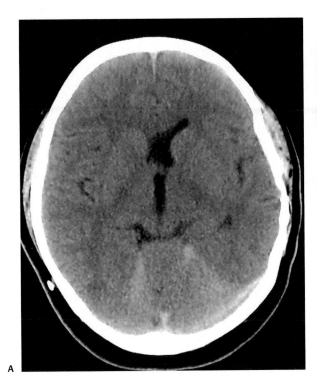

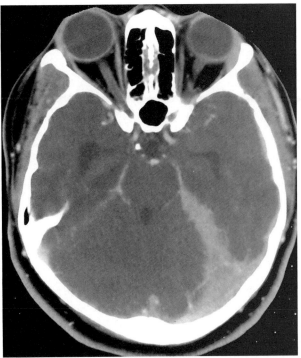

A                                                                                                                    B

## Clinical Presentation

A 17-year-old boy with progression of severe headache and lethargy that started 2 days prior.

### Further Work-up

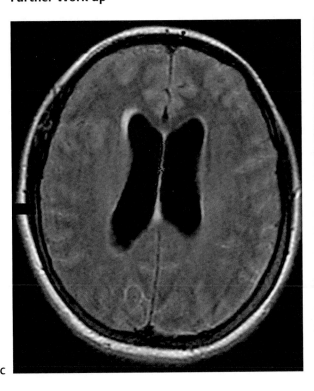

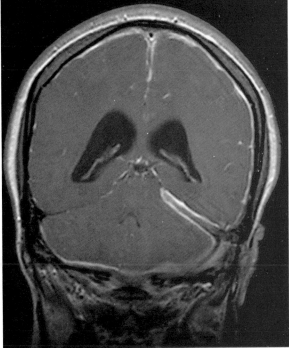

C                                                                                                                    D

## ■ Imaging Findings

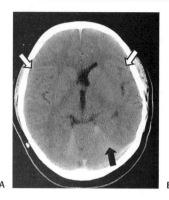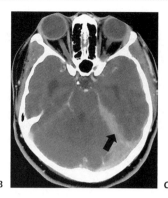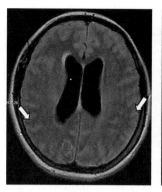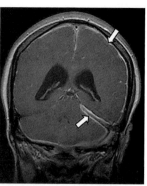

A    B    C    D

**(A)** Computed tomography (CT) without contrast shows effacement of the sulci (*white arrows*) and hyperdensity along the tentorium (*black arrow*). **(B)** CT with contrast shows diffuse meningeal enhancement that is more prominent on the left tentorium (*black arrow*). **(C)** Axial fluid-attenuated inversion recovery (FLAIR) image shows dilated ventricles with increased signal in the leptomeninges (*arrows*). **(D)** Coronal T1-weighted image (WI) with contrast shows diffuse enhancement of the meninges, more prominent on the left side (*arrows*); the ventricles are dilated.

## ■ Differential Diagnosis

- **Bacterial meningitis:** This is infectious leptomeningeal inflammation. Smooth, diffuse enhancement of the pia and arachnoid will be present. Enhancement is thicker in pyogenic meningitis than in viral meningitis. The sulci are effaced. Imaging findings can be normal in the initial phase.
- **Tuberculous meningitis:** Tuberculosis causes granulomatous meningitis. This is usually focal and occurs predominantly in the cisterns around the skull base. There is thickened (nodular) enhancement and possibly parenchymal extension (tuberculomas).
- **Meningeal carcinomatosis:** This is secondary extension of tumors to the meninges. It can affect the dura mater, leptomeninges, or both. The primary lesion can be intra- or extracranial. It can present as smooth or nodular enhancement. In the spine, drop metastases appear as masses or "sugar coating" after contrast administration. It is important to scan the entire neuraxis.

## ■ Essential Facts

- Infectious meningitis can be viral or bacterial.
- Bacterial meningitis secondary to meningococcal infection must be suspected in adolescents and young adults.
- Always use cerebrospinal fluid laboratories to the confirm diagnosis. Parenchymal extension is rare.

## ■ Other Imaging Findings

- CT findings can be normal or show slight leptomeningeal enhancement.
- FLAIR magnetic resonance imaging shows increased leptomeningeal signal; late enhancement makes this finding more conspicuous. T1WIs with contrast will show smooth, diffuse enhancement.

## ✓ Pearls & ✗ Pitfalls

- ✓ Delayed FLAIR images have been shown to be sensitive for leptomeningeal disease if compared with the other magnetic resonance sequences.
- ✗ Increased FLAIR leptomeningeal signal is nonspecific. It has also been described in subarachnoid hemorrhage and stroke, and after general anesthesia.

# Case 71

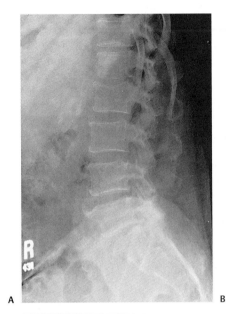

A

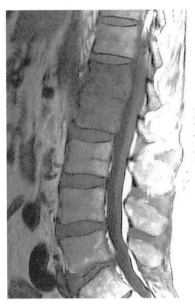

B

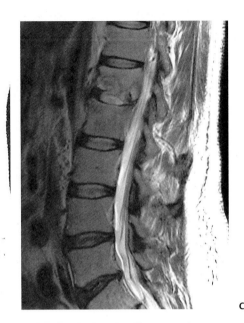

C

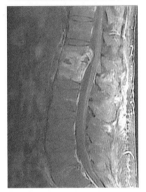

D

## ■ Clinical Presentation

A 59-year-old man with a 1-month history of worsening back pain.

## ■ Imaging Findings

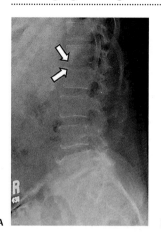
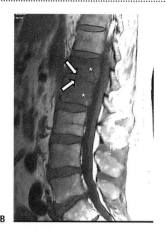
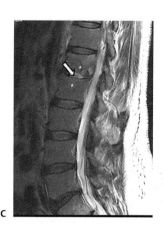
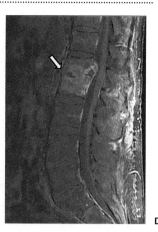

A    B    C    D

**(A)** Lateral view of the lumbar spine shows a decrease of the intervertebral space at L1-2 with poor definition of the adjacent end plates (*arrows*). **(B)** Sagittal T1-weighted image (WI) of the spine shows low signal in the L1 and L2 vertebral bodies (*asterisks*). The L1-2 disk shows low signal with poorly defined adjacent end plates (*arrows*). **(C)** Sagittal T2WI shows increased signal in the L1 and L2 vertebral bodies (*asterisks*) and in the L1-2 disk (*arrows*). **(D)** Sagittal fat-saturated T1WI of the lumbar spine with contrast shows diffuse enhancement of the L1 and L2 vertebral bodies and of the L1-2 disk (*arrow*).

## ■ Differential Diagnosis

- ***Spondylodiskitis:*** This is pyogenic infection of the intervertebral disk and osteomyelitis of the adjacent vertebral bodies. The most frequent pathogen is *Staphylococcus aureus*. The disk and adjacent vertebral bodies enhance.
- *Pott disease:* Tuberculous osteomyelitis is also known as Pott disease. It is a granulomatous infection of the spine that causes large perivertebral abscesses with thin walls and end plate destruction. It involves more than two nonadjacent vertebral bodies, frequently with noncontiguous lesions that skip portions of the vertebral bodies. The midthoracic spine is more often affected than the cervical and lumbar spine.
- *Spinal metastasis:* The spine is the most frequent location for skeletal metastasis. Involvement of the posterior components of the bone is common. Spinal metastasis enhances with contrast and spares the disks.

## ■ Essential Facts

- Ill-defined perivertebral T2 signal abnormality and enhancement are frequent in spondylodiskitis.
- Erosion or destruction of the adjacent end plates occurs in 75% of cases.
- Paraspinal or epidural abscesses with thick walls may be present, although late in the disease.
- Spondylodiskitis usually involves the lumbar spine.
- Subligamentous spread of infection is rare, so there are no "skipped" portions of the vertebral bodies.
- Involvement of more than two vertebral bodies is unusual.

## ■ Other Imaging Findings

- Computed tomography shows normal or decreased density of the vertebral body and end plate destruction.
- On magnetic resonance imaging, the lesion will show low T1 signal of the vertebral body and ill-defined adjacent end plates, with increased T2 signal of the vertebral body and disk. T1 with contrast shows enhancement of the affected segments with disk and diffuse soft-tissue enhancement. If abscess is present, there will be a thick enhancing wall.
- Fluorodeoxyglucose (FDG) positron emission tomography can be helpful to differentiate degenerative from inflammatory end plate changes; degenerative changes do not show FDG uptake.

## ✓ Pearls & ✗ Pitfalls

- ✓ Noninfectious spondylodiskitis is called rheumatic spondylodiskitis and is seen in 8% of patients with ankylosing spondylitis.
- ✗ Tuberculous spondylitis starts in the anterior vertebral body and progresses to the posterior aspects.
- ✗ The disk can be affected late in Pott disease.

# Case 72

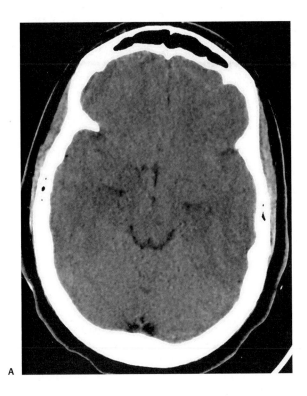

A

## Clinical Presentation

A 37-year-old man with immunosuppression and acute neurologic deficit.

## Further Work-up

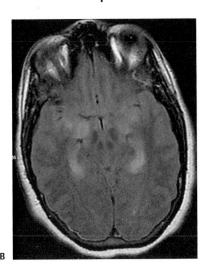

B

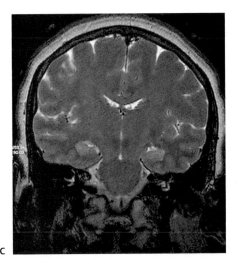

C

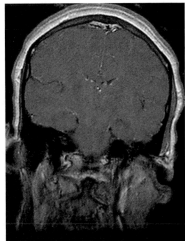

D

### ▪ Imaging Findings

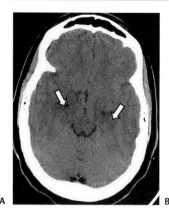
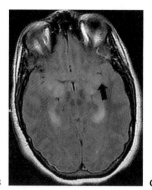
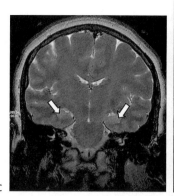
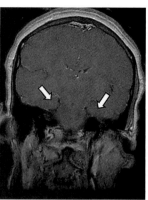

A  B  C  D

**(A)** Axial computed tomography (CT) without contrast shows decreased density of the medial aspect of both temporal lobes (*arrows*). **(B)** Axial fluid-attenuated inversion recovery (FLAIR) image shows high signal in the medial aspect of both temporal lobes with a lack of gray–white matter differentiation (*arrow*). **(C)** Coronal T2-weighted image (WI) of the brain shows increased signal in the medial temporal lobes bilaterally (*arrows*). **(D)** Coronal T1WI of the brain with contrast shows patchy enhancement of the hippocampal region (*arrows*).

### ▪ Differential Diagnosis

- *Herpes encephalitis:* Herpes virus is the most frequent cause of infectious limbic encephalitis, which is characterized by cortical inflammation in the medial aspect of the temporal lobe, high FLAIR signal, loss of gray–white matter differentiation, and restricted diffusion. The onset is usually acute.
- *Autoimmune limbic encephalitis:* Causes may be paraneoplastic (associated with lung, thymus, breast, or testicular cancer) or nonparaneoplastic (rare, associated with voltage-gated potassium channel antibody). Images appear like those of herpes encephalitis, but the acute clinical presentation is lacking. Autoimmune limbic encephalitis involves the limbic system, medial temporal lobe, cingulate gyrus, insula, and inferior frontal lobe. The involved areas show increased T2 and FLAIR signal, with patchy enhancement. There is no mass effect. There is no restriction on diffusion-weighted images (DWIs).
- *Temporal lobe astrocytoma:* This is a unilateral mass in the temporal lobe, with high T2 signal, no enhancement, and no restricted diffusion. The symptoms are not acute.

### ▪ Essential Facts

- The mortality rate is 50 to 70%.
- Herpes encephalitis can progress to necrotizing encephalitis.
- It is more frequent in patients with immunocompromise.
- It can also affect other limbic structures, such as the insula, cingulate gyrus, and inferior frontal lobe.
- It is typically bilateral but can present on only one side.
- Mass effect may be present in the acute phase.

### ▪ Other Imaging Findings

- CT findings can be normal early in the disease; hypodensities in the medial temporal lobes are seen in late disease. CT can detect hemorrhage.
- Magnetic resonance imaging shows loss of gray–white matter differentiation with increased T2/FLAIR signal in the medial temporal lobes involving the cortex. Restricted diffusion on DWIs; can show patchy enhancement with contrast. Gradient-echo imaging can detect hemorrhagic areas.

### ✓ Pearls & ✗ Pitfalls

- ✓ If a focal, well-defined area of enhancement is seen, suspect a malignant tumor.
- ✗ The presentation of congenital herpes simplex virus encephalitis is different from the presentation of herpes encephalitis in adults.

# Case 73

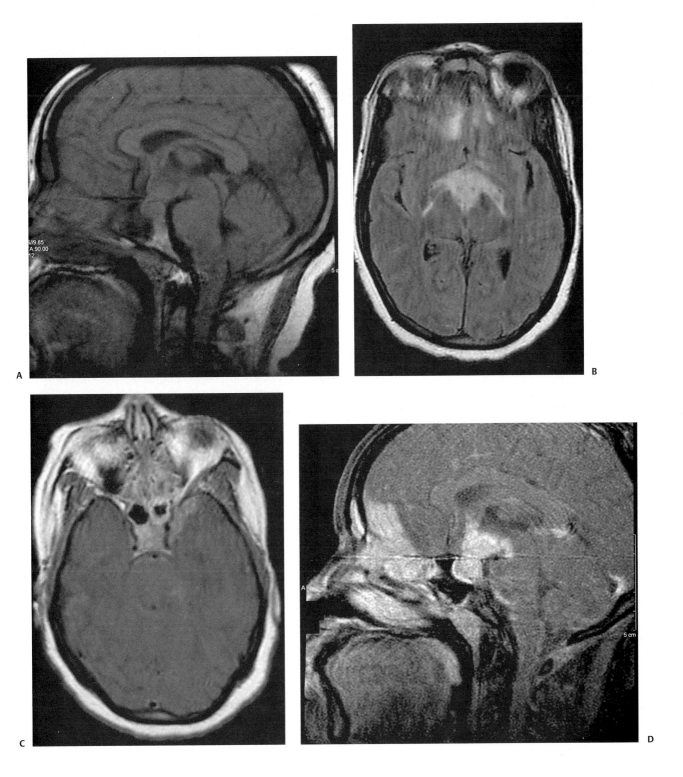

A

B

C

D

## Clinical Presentation

A 37-year-old man with severe headache and palsy of the left abducens nerve.

## Imaging Findings

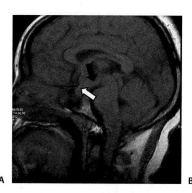 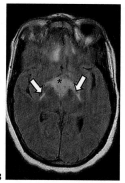 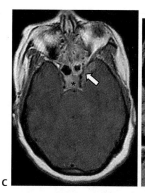 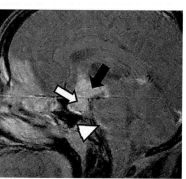

A    B    C    D

**(A)** Sagittal T1-weighted image (WI) shows a thickened pituitary stalk (*white arrow*) with effacement of the infundibulum (*black arrow*). **(B)** Axial fluid-attenuated inversion recovery (FLAIR) image shows high signal in the perimesencephalic cistern (*arrows*) and infundibular region (*asterisk*). There is also increased signal in the frontal lobes. **(C)** Axial T1WI with contrast shows enhancement in the sellar region (*asterisk*) that extends to the cavernous sinus on the left (*arrow*). **(D)** Sagittal T1WI with contrast shows enhancement that involves the sellar region (*white arrow*), infundibulum (*black arrow*), and frontal region. Enhancement is also present in the prepontine cistern (*arrowhead*).

## Differential Diagnosis

- **Tuberculous meningitis:** This is a granulomatous infection of the basilar meninges. It is secondary to lung disease. Imaging shows thick nodular enhancement and associated parenchymal disease (tuberculomas). Tuberculous meningitis has a predilection for the suprasellar region.
- *Meningeal sarcoidosis:* Sarcoidosis causes a granulomatous meningitis with thick nodular enhancement. Less frequently, parenchymal extension through the Virchow-Robin spaces is seen. It can involve the suprasellar region. Disease isolated to cranial nerves or the pituitary stalk is common.
- *Nontuberculous infectious meningitis:* This is leptomeningeal inflammation of viral or bacterial etiology. Meningococcal meningitis affects adolescents and young adults. Smooth, diffuse enhancement of the pia and arachnoid may be present. The sulci are effaced. Imaging findings can be normal in the initial phase. Parenchymal extension is rare.

## Essential Facts

- Tuberculomas can be solid or show thick ring enhancement.
- Parenchymal tuberculomas are secondary to hematogenous spread, typically through the Virchow-Robin spaces, as in cryptococcosis and sarcoidosis.

## Other Imaging Findings

- The results of computed tomography without contrast can be normal; in postcontrast studies, the basal cisterns and tuberculomas enhance.
- On magnetic resonance imaging (MRI), tuberculoma shows low T1 signal and increased T2 signal in the center of the area of necrosis.
- FLAIR image shows increased leptomeningeal signal. T1WI with contrast shows nodular enhancement of the meninges, solid or thick ring enhancement of tuberculoma.

## ✓ Pearls & ✗ Pitfalls

- ✓ Magnetization transfer MRI can help detect early involvement of the meninges in patients with tuberculosis.
- ✓ Consider the diagnosis of histiocytosis in children (4–6 years of age) with pituitary stalk involvement.

# Case 74

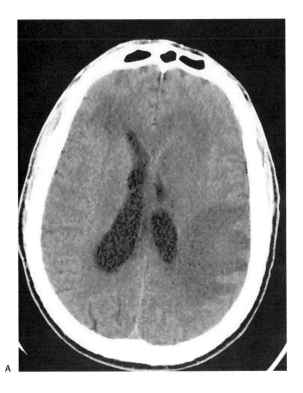

A

## Clinical Presentation

A 42-year-old patient infected with human immunodeficiency virus presenting with deteriorating mental status.

## Further Work-up

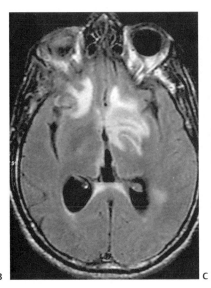

B

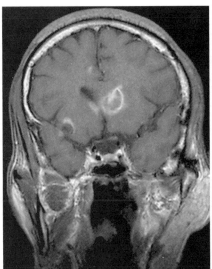

C

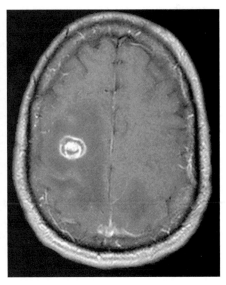

D

### ■ Imaging Findings

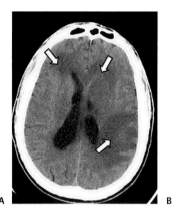
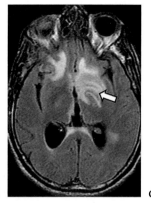
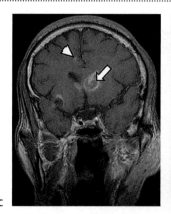
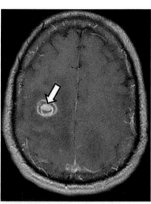

A　　　　　　　　B　　　　　　　　C　　　　　　　　D

**(A)** Computed tomography (CT) of the brain without contrast shows areas of low attenuation in the white matter of both frontal lobes and in the left parietal region (*arrows*) related to vasogenic edema (the cortex is spared). There is effacement of the left frontal horn because of mass effect. **(B)** Axial fluid-attenuated inversion recovery sequence shows high signal in the frontal lobes bilaterally and in the left basal ganglia (*arrow*). **(C)** Coronal T1-weighted image (WI) with contrast shows a lesion with ring enhancement in the head of the left caudate nucleus (*arrow*) and a small enhancing lesion in the gray–white matter junction in the medial right frontal lobe (*arrowhead*). **(D)** Axial magnetic resonance (MR) imaging with contrast shows an "eccentric target sign" in the right frontal lobe. There is a halo of ring enhancement with a nodular enhancing center (*arrow*).

### ■ Differential Diagnosis

- **Toxoplasmosis:** This is the most common mass lesion in patients with acquired immunodeficiency syndrome (AIDS). Multiple lesions with ring enhancement affect the corticomedullary junction and basal ganglia. Toxoplasmosis does not extend to the ependymal surface. Eccentric target sign enhancement is highly suggestive of toxoplasmosis. Acute lesions can have vasogenic edema. Occasional hemorrhage (helps differentiate toxoplasmosis from lymphoma) can be present.
- *Primary central nervous system (CNS) lymphoma:* CNS lymphoma causes basal ganglia and periventricular lesions that enhance. It frequently affects the corpus callosum and can extend to the ependymal surface. Vasogenic edema is less frequent. No hemorrhage should be present.
- *Metastases:* These are usually white–gray matter junction masses. They are solid or necrotic with ring enhancement and vasogenic edema. They are rare in the basal ganglia (3%). Twenty to 50% are solitary lesions.

### ■ Essential Facts

- In adults, most *Toxoplasma gondii* infections are subclinical, but severe infection can occur in patients with immunocompromise, such as those who have AIDS and malignancies.
- Toxoplasmosis is the most common opportunistic CNS infection in patients with AIDS (15–50%).
- Drug therapy does not eradicate *T. gondii*, and lifelong therapy to avoid relapse is often necessary in patients with immunocompromise.

### ■ Other Imaging Findings

- CT shows multiple areas of abnormal hypodensity in the basal ganglia and gray–white matter junction with ring enhancement.
- MR imaging: Lesions are hypo- or isointense on T1WIs and hypo- or isointense with surrounding vasogenic edema on T2WIs. Contrast will show an enhancing ring that can present with a central enhancing nodule (eccentric target sign).

### ✓ Pearls & ✗ Pitfalls

✓ It is extremely difficult to distinguish between toxoplasmosis and lymphoma on imaging. Empiric treatment is usually administered, and the lesions must be followed until they resolve completely.

✓ If there is no improvement after treatment, thallium 201 single-photon emission computed tomography of the brain, positron emission tomography (results of both are positive for lymphoma), or MR spectroscopy can be used to re-evaluate.

✗ Diffusion-weighted and apparent diffusion coefficient lesion: white matter ratios greater than 1.6 favor toxoplasmosis over lymphoma.

# Case 75

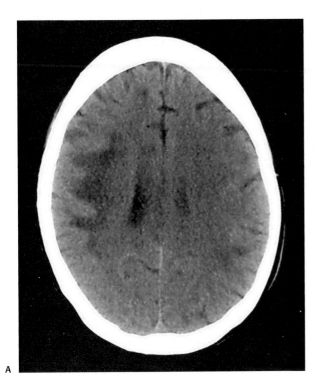

A

## ■ Clinical Presentation

A patient infected with human immunodeficiency virus presenting with headache, hemiparesis, and seizures.

## Further Work-up

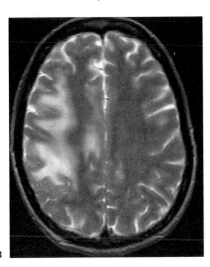

B

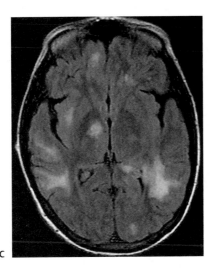

C

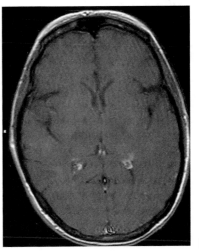

D

### ■ Imaging Findings

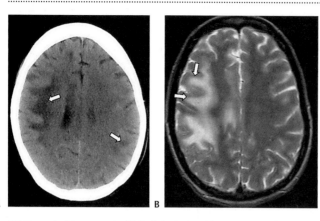
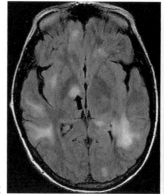
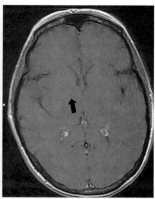

**(A)** Computed tomography (CT) of the brain without contrast shows asymmetric patchy areas of low attenuation bilaterally (*arrows*) with involvement of the subcortical U-fibers. **(B)** Axial T2-weighted image (WI) shows patchy scattered areas of increased intensity bilaterally, more prominent on the right side, involving the subcortical U-fibers (*arrows*). **(C)** Axial fluid-attenuated inversion recovery (FLAIR) image shows multiple patchy areas of hyperintensity involving the subcortical white matter and the right thalamus (*arrow*). **(D)** Magnetic resonance (MR) imaging of the brain with contrast shows no enhancement (*arrow*).

### ■ Differential Diagnosis

- ***Progressive multifocal leukoencephalopathy (PML):*** PML results in diffuse, patchy, asymmetric white matter lesions that are located bilaterally, mainly in the subcortical and periventricular white matter. PML has a predilection for the supratentorial region (parietal and frontal lobes) and thalamus (50% of patients). It spares the cortex and does not show mass effect or contrast enhancement. Cortical atrophy is present in 70% of cases and ventricular dilatation in 50%. PML is hypodense on CT.
- *Human immunodeficiency virus (HIV) encephalitis:* This typically causes cortical atrophy and ventricular dilatation with diffuse, symmetric, periventricular white matter T2 hyperintensities. There is no mass effect. The lesions are confluent and symmetric and do not enhance with contrast. The subcortical white matter is spared.
- *Cytomegalovirus (CMV) infection:* CMV infection causes encephalitis with periventricular white matter hyperintensities and ventriculitis with periventricular enhancement. Imaging findings are nonspecific or absent.

### ■ Essential Facts

- PML is a fulminating opportunistic infection with JC polyomavirus (named for John Cunningham).
- It is a progressive demyelinating disease; the virus targets oligodendrocytes.
- Suspect PML in patients infected with HIV when patchy subcortical high signal appears on T2 or FLAIR.
- The corpus callosum can be involved.

### ■ Other Imaging Findings

- CT shows bilateral asymmetric areas of low attenuation.
- MR imaging: Lesions are hypointense on T1 and hyperintense on T2 and FLAIR. There is no diffusion on diffusion-WIs. MR spectroscopy can detect high levels of choline and variable levels of myoinositol.

### ✓ Pearls & ✗ Pitfalls

- ✓ JC polyomavirus was formerly known as papovirus.
- ✓ Rarely, PML can enhance.
- ✓ The magnetization transfer ratio in PML is severely decreased in comparison with that in HIV encephalitis.
- ✗ Look for involvement of the subcortical U-fibers to favor a diagnosis of PML.

# Case 76

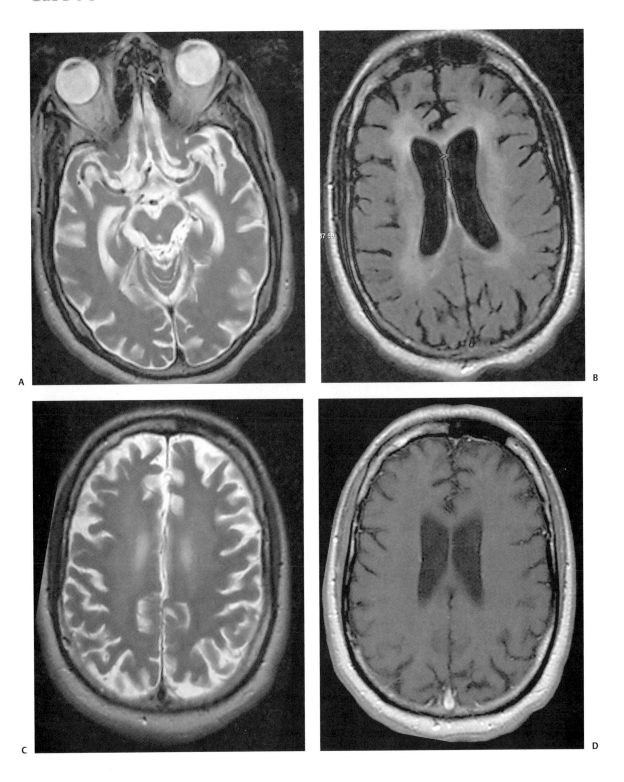

■ **Clinical Presentation**

A 40-year-old man infected with human immunodeficiency virus presenting with progressive dementia and tremor.

■ **Imaging Findings**

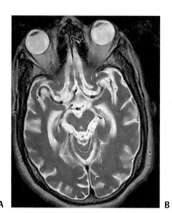
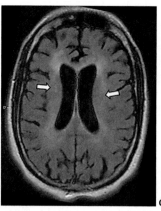
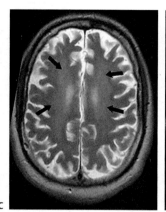
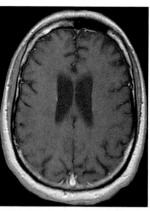

A     B     C     D

**(A)** Axial T2-weighted image (WI) shows diffuse cerebral atrophy. **(B)** Axial fluid-attenuated inversion recovery (FLAIR) image shows diffuse cerebral atrophy with symmetric, confluent periventricular white matter disease (*arrows*). The subcortical white matter is spared. **(C)** Axial T2WI shows the symmetric periventricular white matter hyperintensities (*arrows*), with sparing of the subcortical U-fibers. **(D)** Axial T1WI with contrast shows no enhancement of the periventricular lesions.

■ **Differential Diagnosis**

- ***Human immunodeficiency virus (HIV) encephalopathy:*** This is characterized by cortical atrophy, ventricular dilatation, and diffuse periventricular white matter T2 hyperintensities that are confluent and symmetric. The subcortical white matter is spared. It appears hypodense on computed tomography (CT). There is no enhancement or mass effect.
- *Progressive multifocal leukoencephalopathy (PML):* Diffuse, patchy, asymmetric white matter lesions are located bilaterally, mainly in the subcortical and periventricular white matter. Involvement of the subcortical U-fibers is common. The lesions have a predilection for the supratentorial region (parietal and frontal lobes). Cortical atrophy and ventricular dilatation are less frequent. There is no mass effect or enhancement.
- *Cytomegalovirus (CMV) infection:* Imaging is nonspecific, and findings can be normal. Encephalitis with periventricular white matter hyperintensities is common. Ventriculitis with periventricular enhancement is characteristic. CMV encephalitis is a rapidly advancing disease (progression is faster than in HIV leukoencephalitis) that leads to death, usually in 5 to 8 weeks.

■ **Essential Facts**

- HIV encephalopathy is the most common neurologic disease of the central nervous system caused by the HIV itself.
- Others include vacuolar myelopathy, peripheral neuropathies, and polymyositis.
- HIV causes diffuse myelin loss and astroglial proliferation by mono- and multinuclear macrophages.
- There is frontal dominance. The genu of the corpus callosum may be involved.

■ **Other Imaging Findings**

- CT shows atrophy with confluent periventricular low-density lesions; there is no enhancement.
- Magnetic resonance (MR) imaging: Lesions are iso- or hypointense on T1 and hyperintense on T2/FLAIR. They show no enhancement.
  - MR spectroscopy shows high myoinositol and choline levels and reduced *N*-acetyl aspartate levels.

✓ **Pearls & ✗ Pitfalls**

- ✓ The magnetization transfer ratio in PML is severely decreased in comparison with that in HIV encephalitis.
- ✗ The presence of ependymal enhancement favors CMV.
- ✗ HIV leukoencephalitis does not present with mass effect or enhancement.
- ✗ In the late stages of HIV leukoencephalopathy, the lesions can involve all the white matter, including the subcortical fibers.

# Case 77

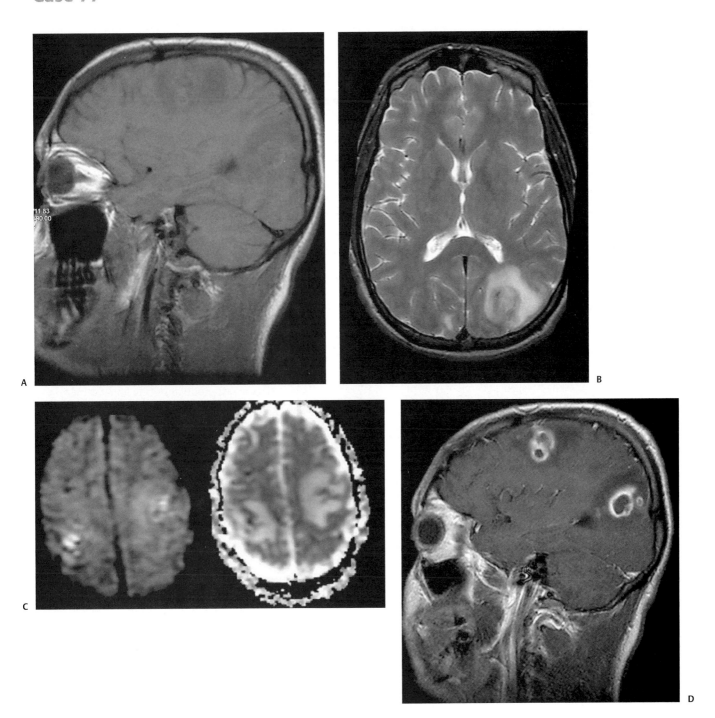

A

B

C

D

## Clinical Presentation

A 39-year-old drug addict with heart disease.

## Imaging Findings

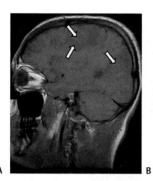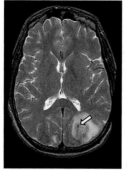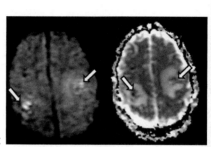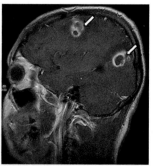

A    B    C    D

**(A)** Sagittal T1-weighted image (WI) shows heterogeneous subcortical nodules (*arrows*) surrounded by areas of low intensity related to vasogenic edema. The walls demonstrate areas of hyperintensity related to bleeding. **(B)** Axial T2WI shows vasogenic edema in the left occipital lobe with a central nodular area. There is an area of low signal in the lesion that is related to the bleed (*arrow*). **(C)** Diffusion-WI and apparent diffusion coefficient map show bilateral areas of restricted diffusion (*arrows*). **(D)** Sagittal T1WI with contrast shows subcortical lesions with ring enhancement (*arrows*).

## Differential Diagnosis

- **Septic emboli:** Hematogenous dissemination of septic emboli may result from cardiac valvular disease. The lesions are usually in the territory of the middle cerebral artery (MCA) and are predominantly subcortical. Restricted diffusion, hemorrhage, and nodular or ring enhancement are common. Surrounding vasogenic edema may be present.
- *Metastasis:* Hematogenous metastasis occurs in the cortical or subcortical white matter, frequently in the territory of the MCA. Surrounding vasogenic edema is characteristic. There is no restricted diffusion. Hemorrhage and nodular or ring enhancement may be present. A known primary tumor makes this diagnosis more likely.
- *Aseptic emboli:* Aseptic emboli are bilateral or unilateral small infarcts in the subcortical white matter without hemorrhage. They often occur in the territory of the MCA. There is no surrounding vasogenic edema, enhancement, or hemorrhage. Emboli may arise in the heart or large vessels, usually at the carotid bifurcation.

## Essential Facts

- Endocarditis must be suspected.
- Echocardiography and blood cultures are a part of the work-up.
- *Staphylococcus aureus* and *Streptococcus viridans* are the most common pathogens.
- In intravenous (IV) drug abusers, *Staphylococcus* infection and fungal septic emboli can occur.

## Other Imaging Findings

- Computed tomography shows punctate areas of hypodensity that are hyperdense if hemorrhage is present.
- MRI:
  - T1WIs: small areas of low signal
  - T2WIs: vasogenic edema around a hyperintense lesion
  - T1WIs with contrast: nodular or ring enhancement
  - Diffusion-WIs: restricted diffusion
  - Gradient-echo images: blooming in areas of hemorrhage

## ✓ Pearls & ✗ Pitfalls

- ✓ Hemorrhage is commonly associated with septic emboli.
- ✓ In IV drug abusers with intracranial hemorrhage, a study of the intracranial vasculature to exclude mycotic aneurysms is recommended.
- ✗ Diffusion-WIs and IV contrast can help to differentiate between tumoral (no restriction, enhancement) and nontumoral (restriction, no enhancement) emboli to the brain.

# Case 78

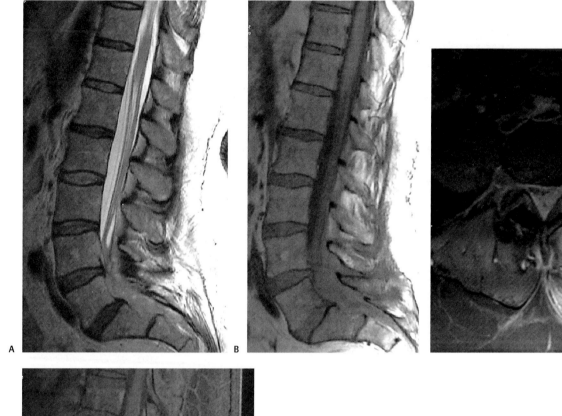

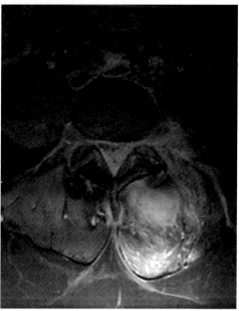

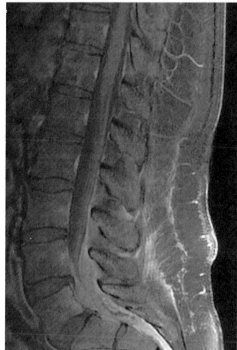

## ■ Clinical Presentation

A patient with increased radicular pain and fever 1 month after laminectomy.

### ■ Imaging Findings

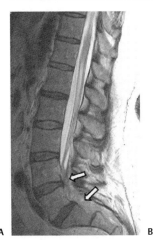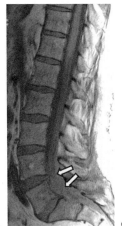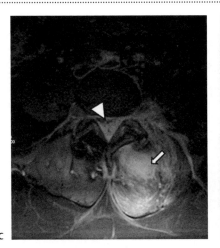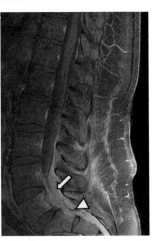

**(A)** Sagittal T2-weighted image (WI) shows heterogeneous signal in the lower lumbar spine (*arrows*). **(B)** Sagittal T1WI shows isointense signal in the lower lumbar spinal canal (*arrows*); the nerve roots are not seen. **(C)** Fat-saturated axial T1WI with contrast shows enhancement of the left paraspinal muscles and the posterior aspect of the spinal canal (*arrow*) compressing the thecal sac (*arrowhead*). **(D)** Fat-saturated T1WI of the lumbar spine with contrast shows concentric anterior and posterior enhancement of the epidural space (*arrow*) and a central area without enhancement (*arrowhead*).

### ■ Differential Diagnosis

- *Epidural abscess:* This is an infectious collection outside the dura mater that can be associated with osteomyelitis or paraspinal infection. Epidural abscess usually extends along two to nine vertebral segments. It demonstrates increased T2 signal in the epidural space compressing the thecal sac. There is avid enhancement and a thick capsule. Diffusely increased T2 signal of the paraspinal soft tissues is noted.
- *Epidural hemorrhage:* This is characterized by a fluid collection outside the dura mater with variable signal intensity depending on the age of the hemorrhage. It usually extends beyond three consecutive vertebral segments. Epidural hemorrhage can have marginal enhancement.
- *Epidural tumor:* Epidural metastases are usually an extension of vertebral body lesions. Neurofibromas or schwannomas can occupy the epidural space, but they are commonly fusiform or dumbbell-shaped masses confined to one vertebral level and adjacent to the neural foramen.

### ■ Essential Facts

- The primary source of infection is usually the vertebral body or disk, followed by the joint facet and perivertebral soft tissues.
- The center of the abscess shows fluid signal with thick peripheral enhancement.

### ■ Other Imaging Findings

- Computed tomography results can be normal. Look for findings of primary infection.
- Magnetic resonance imaging:
  - T1WIs: The center is isointense to hypointense. If the protein level of the abscess contents is high, T1WIs can show increased signal.
  - T2WIs: The signal is heterogeneous, mostly increased. There is diffuse high signal in the adjacent soft tissues.
  - T1WIs with contrast show avid enhancement of the walls.

### ✓ Pearls & ✗ Pitfalls

- ✓ Diffusion-WIs can help differentiate abscess from hematoma.
- ✗ The signal intensity of cerebrospinal fluid can be similar to that of abscess, making abscess difficult to detect on T2WIs.

# Case 79

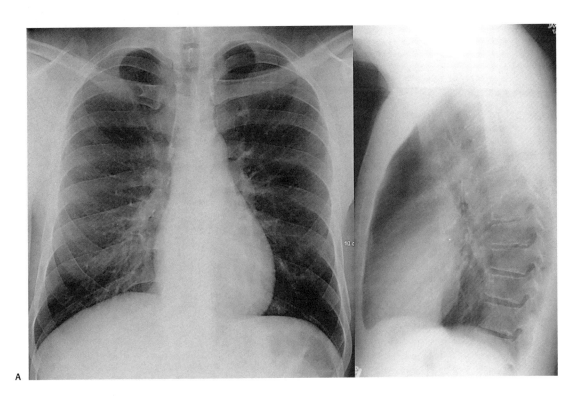

A

## Clinical Presentation

A 45-year-old patient with chronic cough who is now experiencing persistent back pain.

## Further Work-up

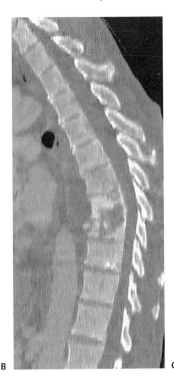

B

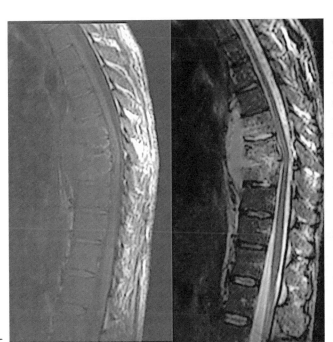

C

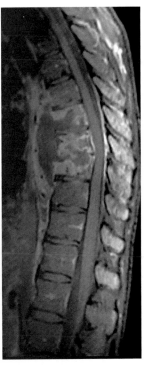

D

### ■ Imaging Findings

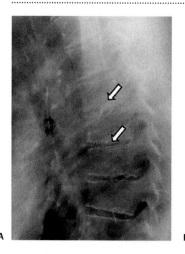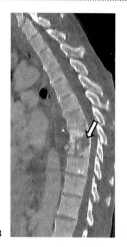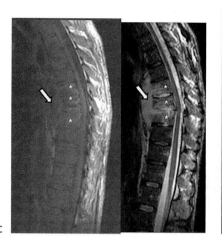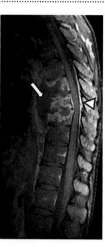

A    B    C    D

**(A)** Lateral radiograph of the thoracic spine shows irregular end plates and narrowed disk spaces of the midthoracic vertebrae (*arrows*). **(B)** Sagittal reformatted computed tomography (CT) of the thoracic spine without contrast shows hypodense destructive changes of a vertebra (*arrow*). There is a prevertebral collection (*asterisk*). **(C)** Sagittal T1- and T2-weighted images (WIs) of the thoracic spine show low T1 and high T2 signal of three adjacent vertebral bodies (*asterisks*). There is an anterior well-defined fluid collection with a thin capsule adjacent to these segments (*arrows*). **(D)** Fat-saturated sagittal T1WI of the thoracic spine with contrast shows enhancement of the three thoracic segments and rim enhancement of the fluid collection (*arrow*). There is a small area of posterior epidural enhancement (*arrowhead*).

### ■ Differential Diagnosis

- **Tuberculous spondylitis:** Also known as Pott disease, tuberculous spondylitis has a predilection for the upper lumbar and lower thoracic spine. More than one vertebral body is usually involved. The disk is compromised late in the disease and may appear collapsed. Anterior wedging leads to gibbous deformity. There is usually early paravertebral abscess formation with a thin wall. Subligamentous spread of the infection affects three or more levels. Soft-tissue calcifications may be present.
- *Pyogenic spondylodiskitis:* This is bacterial infection of the disk and vertebral body. It is more frequent in the lower lumbar or cervical spine. Pyogenic spondylodiskitis has a thick, irregular abscess wall. There is involvement of the intervertebral disk and the two adjacent vertebral bodies. Erosion of the end plates is typically seen.
- *Spinal metastasis:* Vertebral metastases involve multiple vertebral bodies, including the posterior elements. The disks are not affected. Contrast enhancement is variable.

### ■ Essential Facts

- The upper lumbar spine and lower thoracic spine are the most frequent sites for skeletal involvement of tuberculosis (TB).
- The disease starts in the anterior body adjacent to the end plate and progresses toward the posterior body.
- TB initially shows hematogenous seeding to the anterior vertebral body and then spreads to distant vertebral bodies through the anterior longitudinal ligament.

### ■ Other Imaging Findings

- CT shows destruction of the end plates and soft-tissue calcification.
- Magnetic resonance imaging shows low T1 signal intensity in the affected body and increased T2 signal in the affected body, abscess, and disk. There is enhancement of the vertebral body and abscess.

### ✓ Pearls & ✗ Pitfalls

- ✓ It is essential to evaluate for cord compression resulting from epidural extension of the abscess.
- ✓ In a patient with vertebral body lesions and soft-tissue abscess, look for pulmonary findings of TB.
- ✗ Systemic coccidioidomycosis can present with miliary disease and vertebral osteomyelitis, mimicking TB.

# Case 80

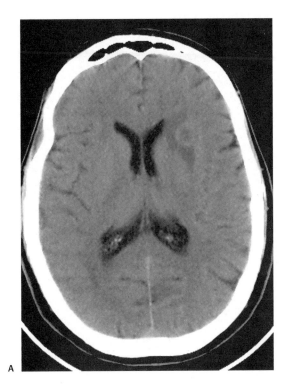

A

## ■ Clinical Presentation

A 36-year-old woman with a history of heroin use presenting with diffuse headache, fever, and seizures.

## Further Work-up

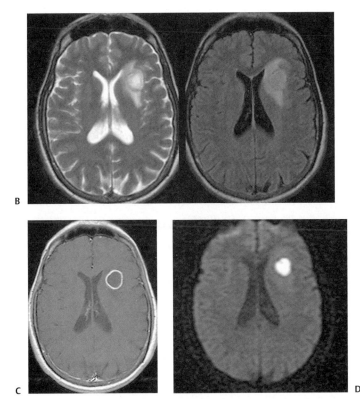

B

C

D

### ■ Imaging Findings

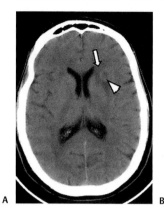
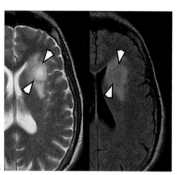
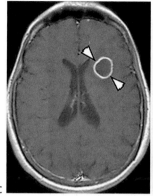
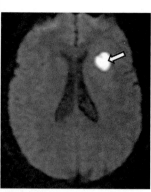

A   B   C   D

**(A)** Axial computed tomography (CT) without contrast shows a ring isodense to the gray matter (*arrowhead*) in the left frontal lobe. The lesion, located at the gray–white matter junction, has a hypodense center and is surrounded by vasogenic edema (*arrow*). **(B)** Axial T2-weighted image (WI) and fluid-attenuated inversion recovery image show the left frontal lesion with a rim of low intensity (*arrowheads*) and peripheral vasogenic edema. **(C)** Axial T1WI with contrast shows a round, well-defined, ring-enhancing lesion in the left frontal lobe (*arrowheads*). The inner and outer margins are smooth. **(D)** Diffusion-WI shows a "lightbulb" sign of the left frontal lesion (*arrow*).

### ■ Differential Diagnosis

- **Cerebral abscess:** This is the organized, late phase of a brain infection. A bacterial etiology is the most common. The gray–white matter junction in the territory of the middle cerebral artery is the most frequent location because of hematogenous spread. A ring-enhancing lesion is described as having smooth inner and outer margins. There is surrounding edema. The lesion presents as high signal on diffusion-WIs with a dark apparent diffusion coefficient (ADC) map.
- **Metastasis:** A hematogenous metastasis involves the cortical or subcortical white matter and occurs more frequently in the territory of the middle cerebral artery. The lesion demonstrates surrounding vasogenic edema, no restricted diffusion, and nodular or ring enhancement. Hemorrhage may be present. A known primary tumor increases the likelihood of this diagnosis.
- **Glioblastoma multiforme:** This is the most common of the primary intracranial neoplasms. The usual presentation is thick, irregular ring enhancement with a serrated inner margin. There is a necrotic center with surrounding edema. The corpus callosum can be affected. Glioblastoma multiforme can have increased signal on diffusion-WIs but usually has no restriction on the ADC map.

### ■ Essential Facts

- Bacterial infection of the brain evolves from cerebritis to capsule formation.
- Abscesses form when a capsule of granulation tissue, reinforced by a collagen wall, confines the infected area of brain and pus.
- Pathogens may enter the brain by hematogenous spread or direct extension of an infection (from the sinuses, mastoid processes, or ears). They may also be introduced following penetrating injury or surgery.

### ■ Other Imaging Findings

- CT: The capsule appears as an isodense rim around a hypodense center with surrounding hypodense edema. The capsule enhances with contrast.
- Magnetic resonance imaging:
  - T2WIs: the rim of an abscess is hypointense; this finding is the first to disappear after treatment.
  - Diffusion-WIs: there is restricted diffusion with restriction on ADC maps.
- Spectroscopy shows increased levels of acetate, alanine and other amino acids, and lactate.

### ✓ Pearls & ✗ Pitfalls

- ✓ In the early phases of transition between cerebritis and an organized abscess, the margins of the capsule can be poorly defined.
- ✓ Highly cellular tumors with areas of necrosis may show restricted diffusion that affects the solid (enhancing) component of the tumor, whereas in abscesses, the restriction involves the pus-filled (nonenhancing) cavity.
- ✗ Extension to the corpus callosum is rare in abscesses.
- ✗ An abscess can rupture through the ependymal lining of the ventricle and cause ventriculitis.
- ✗ Always look for additional lesions.

# Case 81

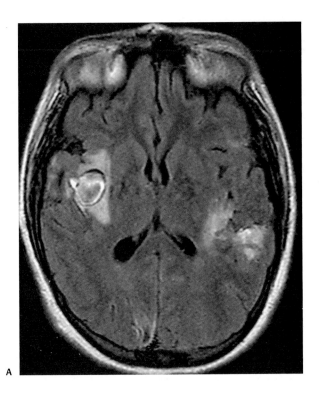

A

## Clinical Presentation

A 35-year-old drug addict with bacterial endocarditis presenting with the sudden onset of severe, worsening headache.

## Further Work-up

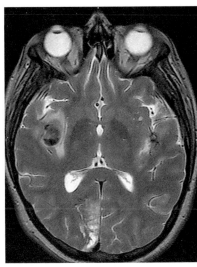

B

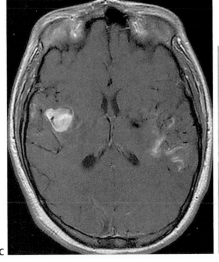

C

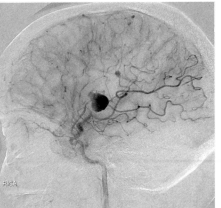

D

## ■ Imaging Findings

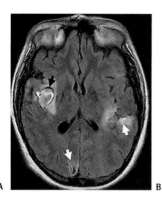
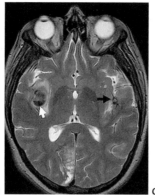
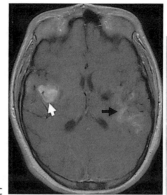
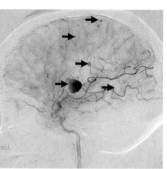

A          B          C          D

**(A)** Axial fluid-attenuated inversion recovery image shows a round lesion in the deep sylvian fissure on the right (*black arrow*) surrounded by vasogenic edema. The lesion has a well-defined capsule of low intensity. Additional hyperintensities are seen in the perisylvian cortex on the left and in the right occipital lobe (*white arrows*). **(B)** Axial T2-weighted image (WI) shows a hypointense round lesion in the deep sylvian fissure on the right (*white arrow*) and a smaller contralateral lesion (*black arrow*). **(C)** Axial T1WI with contrast shows diffuse enhancement of the right sylvian lesion (*white arrow*). There is cortical enhancement in the cortex surrounding the left sylvian fissure (*black arrow*) and in the left occipital lobe. **(D)** Lateral digital subtraction angiography (DSA) of the head in a late arterial phase of the right internal carotid artery injection shows multiple aneurysms throughout the middle cerebral artery (MCA); most are in the distal branches (*arrows*).

## ■ Differential Diagnosis

- **Mycotic aneurysm:** Mycotic aneurysms account for 5% of intracranial aneurysms and are of infectious etiology. Multiple aneurysms are usually present bilaterally, involving the distal segments and unrelated to the branching sites. They can be fusiform. Rapid morphologic changes over time are not uncommon. Mycotic aneurysms are associated with nearby arterial occlusion or stenosis.
- *Saccular aneurysm:* Saccular aneurysms have a "berry" shape. They are located at branching points in the vessels of the circle of Willis. They are unusual in peripheral branches. They can be multiple and are more frequent in females. Ninety percent occur in the anterior circulation.
- *Noninfectious fusiform aneurysm:* These are rare and tend to be large. They form spontaneously and are not related to the bifurcation of vessels. They are not multiple or bilateral.

## ■ Essential Facts

- Vessel wall necrosis after bacterial or fungal embolization results in the formation of multiple intracranial infectious aneurysms.
- Bacterial endocarditis is the most common cause.
- Mycotic aneurysms involve distal branches, typically in the distribution of the MCA.
- They can bleed, and subarachnoid hemorrhage or parenchymal hematoma may develop.
- They can regress after the treatment of endocarditis.
- Endovascular treatment has been proposed for large mycotic aneurysms because of the likelihood of rupture.

## ■ Other Imaging Findings

- Computed tomography (CT) is the initial study of choice if intracranial bleeding is suspected.
- Magnetic resonance (MR) imaging is good for detecting parenchymal hemorrhage and ischemia; however, it can miss small lesions.
- DSA is the imaging gold standard for the detection of the multiple infectious aneurysms; MR angiography and CT angiography are less sensitive.

## ✓ Pearls & ✗ Pitfalls

- ✓ The mortality rates are 32% for bacterial and 90% for fungal infectious aneurysms.
- ✓ The gold standard for the diagnosis is histologic confirmation.
- ✗ Mycotic aneurysms can be round and difficult to differentiate from "berry" aneurysms based solely on their morphology.
- ✗ A history of endocarditis and a positive blood culture are part of the clinical criteria to confirm the diagnosis.

# Case 82

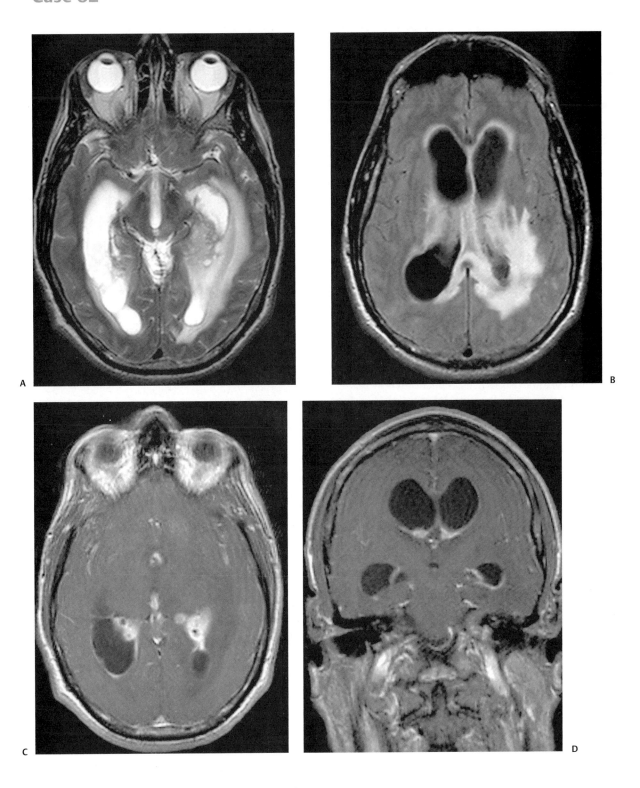

## Clinical Presentation

A 38-year-old man with severe headache and fever.

### ■ Imaging Findings

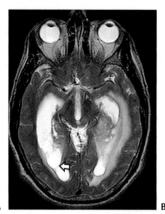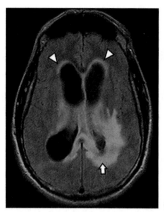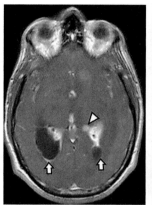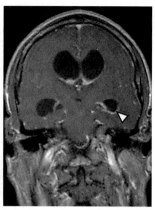

**(A)** Axial T2-weighted image (WI) shows dilated lateral ventricles with a septum in the right occipital horn (*arrow*). **(B)** Axial fluid-attenuated inversion recovery (FLAIR) image shows hyperintense signal around the ventricles (*arrowheads*) that is more prominent around the right atrium (*arrow*). **(C)** Axial T1WI of the brain with contrast shows enhancement at the ependymal lining (*arrows*). There is an enhancing nodule (*arrowhead*) in the left thalamic region. **(D)** Coronal T1WI with contrast shows enhancement of the ventricular wall (*arrowhead*). Note the dilatation of the lateral ventricles.

### ■ Differential Diagnosis

- **Ventriculitis:** Ventriculitis is inflammation of the ependymal lining. Pyogenic infection is the most common cause. If there are pus collections within the ventricles, imaging studies will show bacterial debris, hydrocephalus, symmetric enhancement of the ventricular walls, and restricted diffusion. Seventy-five percent of cases are associated with meningitis.
- *Ventricular extension of tumor:* Primary tumors (usually glioblastoma multiforme) extending to the ventricles will cause T2 signal abnormality in the periventricular region and ependymal enhancement. The enhancement is typically asymmetric. No ventricular debris should be present.
- *Lymphoma:* Ventricular extension of an intracranial lymphoma is one of the characteristics that allows clinicians to differentiate lymphoma from toxoplasmosis in patients infected with human immunodeficiency virus. Imaging will show nodular ependymal enhancement, basal ganglia lesions, and ring-enhancing subcortical lesions. There may be meningeal thickening of the basal cisterns. Isolated ventricular disease without parenchymal disease is extremely rare.

### ■ Essential Facts

- Ventriculitis has a high mortality rate (> 50%).
- Ventricular debris is the most common imaging finding in pyogenic ventriculitis.
- Hydrocephalus develops very rapidly.

### ■ Other Imaging Findings

- Computed tomography shows ventriculomegaly and a fluid level in the ventricle.
- Magnetic resonance imaging: Debris may be hyperintense on T1WIs, with periventricular low signal on T1 and increased signal on T2/FLAIR sequences. The debris and parenchymal abscesses show restricted diffusion. Enhancement of ependymal, meningeal, and parenchymal lesions can be seen.

### ✓ Pearls & ✗ Pitfalls

- ✓ The most common causes of ventriculitis include ventricular catheter infection and ruptured abscess.
- ✓ FLAIR images are superior to postcontrast T1WIs for detecting ventricular wall abnormalities.
- ✗ In trauma patients, ventricular hemorrhage can show increased FLAIR signal in the ependymal lining with obstructive hydrocephalus.

# Case 83

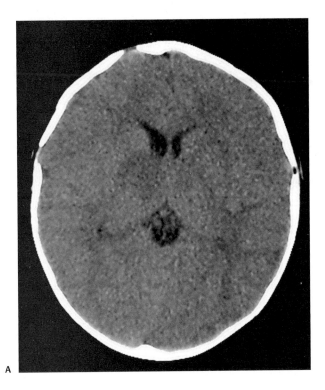

A

## Clinical Presentation

A 1-year-old with altered mental status and seizures following a viral illness.

## Further Work-up

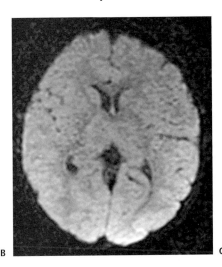

B

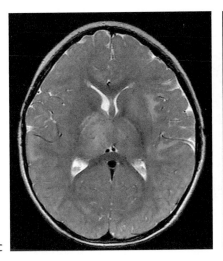

C

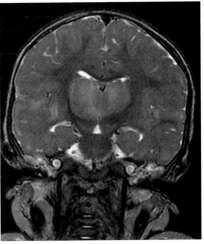

D

### ■ Imaging Findings

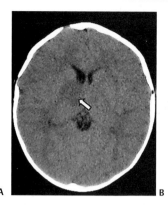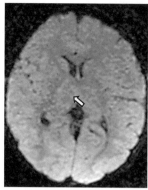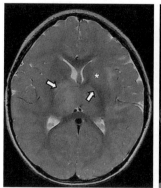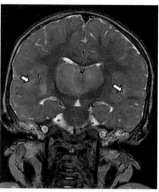

A   B   C   D

**(A)** Axial computed tomography (CT) shows low attenuation in the right thalamus and posterior limb of the internal capsule (*arrow*). **(B)** Axial diffusion-weighted image (WI) fails to show restriction in the right thalamus (*arrow*). **(C)** Axial T2WI demonstrates increased signal intensity in the thalami, internal capsules (*arrows*), lenticular nucleus on the left (*asterisk*), and subcortical white matter bilaterally. **(D)** Coronal T2WI shows enlargement and increased signal in the thalami. There is also increased signal in the subcortical white matter bilaterally (*arrows*).

### ■ Differential Diagnosis

- *Acute disseminated encephalomyelitis (ADEM):* ADEM is a monophasic demyelinating disease of the central nervous system that presents with numerous hyperintense white and gray matter lesions on T2WIs. It has an asymmetric distribution and is poorly marginated. Contrast enhancement is infrequent.
- *Multiple sclerosis (MS):* MS presents with multiple, well-marginated lesions that have a predilection for the periventricular regions and corpus callosum. When the cord is involved, partial myelopathy is present.
- *Viral encephalitis:* This causes the acute onset of a febrile illness and neurologic signs (seizures, alteration of consciousness, meningeal irritation). On magnetic resonance imaging (MRI), there is a variable appearance on diffusion-WIs and T2WIs. Different viruses prefer specific areas: herpes encephalitis favors the medial temporal lobes, Japanese encephalitis is found in the gray matter, and enterovirus 71 favors the rhombencephalon. CT and MRI may show complications such as hemorrhage, hydrocephalus, and herniation.

### ■ Essential Facts

- ADEM presents as multiple gray and white matter lesions of the brain and spinal cord.
- A prior infectious episode or vaccination triggers the inflammatory response.
- Young and adolescent children are most affected.
- The severity of the clinical symptoms is variable; these include seizures, coma, behavioral disturbances, headaches, vomiting, fever, drowsiness, and/or focal neurologic signs.
- Selective involvement of the cerebral cortex may be the only manifestation of ADEM.

- Infratentorial lesions occur in more than 50% of cases (brainstem, middle cerebellar peduncles, and cerebellar white matter).
- ADEM has a favorable prognosis.

### ■ Other Imaging Findings

- CT findings are frequently normal.
- MRI: T2WIs and fluid-attenuated inversion recovery images show multiple, asymmetrically distributed, poorly marginated hyperintense areas involving the white matter and the deep gray matter nuclei (i.e., thalamus and basal ganglia). Contrast enhancement is infrequent. When present, it typically involves the vast majority of lesions simultaneously.

### ✓ Pearls & ✗ Pitfalls

- ✓ Restricted diffusion does not imply irreversible damage in ADEM.
- ✓ Approximately 30% of patients who have ADEM also have lesions in their spinal cord.
- ✗ The neuroradiologic findings of ADEM are not specific and typically do not allow ADEM to be differentiated from MS or encephalitis.

# Case 84

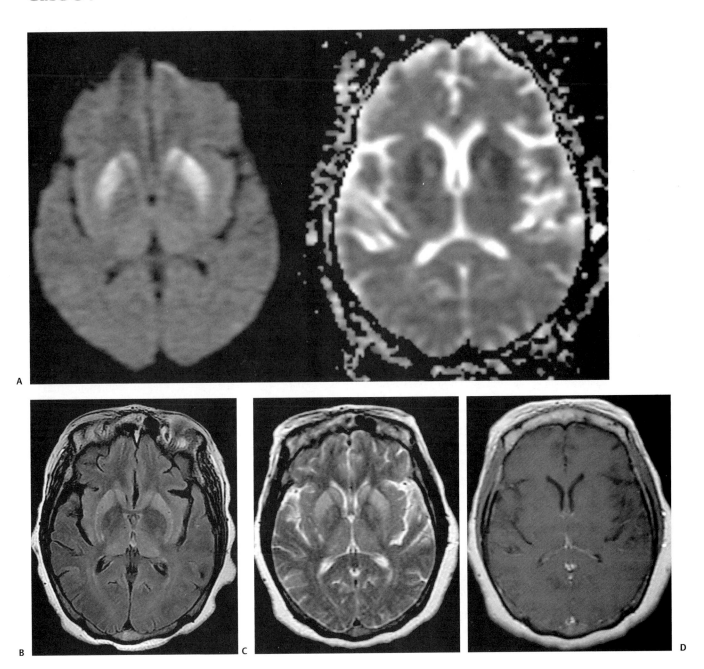

## ■ Clinical Presentation

A 45-year-old woman with rapidly progressive dementia.

## ■ Imaging Findings

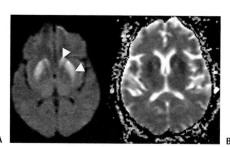
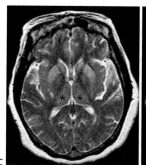
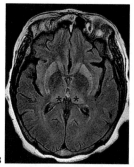
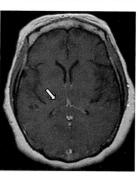

**(A)** Axial diffusion-weighted image (WI) and apparent diffusion coefficient map show areas of restriction in the caudate head and lenticular nuclei (*arrowheads*). **(B)** Axial fluid-attenuated inversion recovery magnetic resonance imaging (MRI) shows symmetric areas of increased T2 signal in the basal ganglia and thalami (*asterisks*). **(C)** Axial T2WI shows symmetric areas of increased T2 signal in the basal ganglia as well as in the thalami (*asterisks*). **(D)** Axial T1WI after gadolinium injection shows no enhancement (*arrow*).

## ■ Differential Diagnosis

- **Creutzfeldt-Jakob disease (CJD):** Symmetric areas of restricted diffusion and T2 hyperintensity involving the basal ganglia in a patient without acute alteration of mental status are highly suggestive of CJD. The lesions do not show mass effect or enhancement.
- *Hypoxic ischemic injury:* This presents clinically as acute alteration of mental status after an episode of cerebral hypoperfusion. Restricted diffusion and T2 signal changes in the basal ganglia and cerebral cortex are found on MRI. There is a predilection for the globus pallidus.
- *Carbon monoxide poisoning:* This is a combination of tissue hypoxia and direct carbon monoxide–mediated damage at the cellular level. Clinically, it may manifest acutely or produce a delayed neurologic syndrome. On MRI, necrosis in the globus pallidus and other basal ganglia is seen as low T1 and high T2 signal; hemorrhage will show high T1 and T2 signal. Carbon monoxide poisoning may also involve the white matter (predominantly periventricular) and cerebral cortex (with a predilection for the medial temporal lobes).

## ■ Essential Facts

- CJD is a prion infectious disease characterized by progressive dementia, other neurologic abnormalities, and eventually death.
- Prions (proteinaceous infectious particles) are infective agents consisting of protein. They lack nucleic acid.
- CJD causes varying degrees of spongiform neuronal degeneration, neuronal loss, reactive astrocytic gliosis, and amyloid-like plaques that predominantly affect gray matter structures.
- There are different subtypes: sporadic, familial, and acquired.
- The clinical presentation includes rapidly progressive dementia, motor dysfunction, myoclonus, and, in the later stages, akinetic mutism and death.

## ■ Other Imaging Findings

- MRI:
  - Symmetric T2 hyperintensity involving the basal ganglia, in particular the corpus striatum
  - Less commonly, asymmetric striatal involvement and signal abnormality in the thalamus and periaqueductal gray matter; cerebral cortical signal abnormality that is either symmetric or asymmetric
  - No mass effect or enhancement
  - Progression to atrophy in the terminal stages
- At magnetic resonance spectroscopy, *N*-acetyl aspartate may be decreased in the early stage of disease.
- Single-photon emission computed tomography performed with technetium 99m–ethyl cysteinate dimer has been reported to show decreased cerebral blood flow in the regions of the brain that correspond to areas with abnormally high signal intensities on diffusion-WIs.

## ✓ Pearls & ✗ Pitfalls

- ✓ MRI findings can precede the onset of characteristic clinical disease, particularly with the use of diffusion-WIs.
- ✗ The pulvinar sign (symmetric high signal in the pulvinar compared with the signal in the remainder of the basal ganglia) is also seen occasionally with other diseases, such as limbic encephalitis.

# Case 85

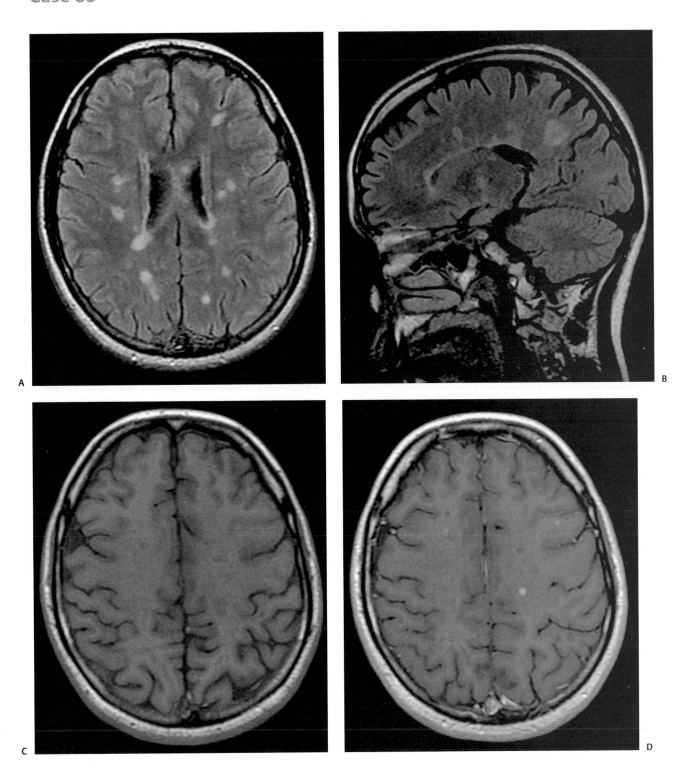

A

B

C

D

## Clinical Presentation

A 30-year-old with headache, weakness, and optic neuritis.

## ■ Imaging Findings

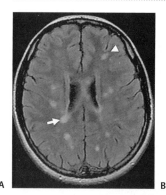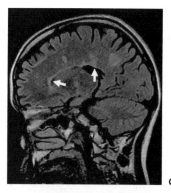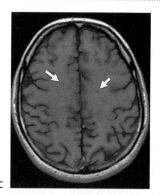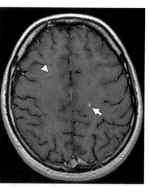

A    B    C    D

**(A)** Axial fluid-attenuated inversion recovery (FLAIR) image shows numerous round and oval areas of increased signal in the periventricular (*arrow*) and subcortical (*arrowhead*) white matter. **(B)** Sagittal FLAIR image demonstrates involvement of the transcallosal white matter tracts (*arrows*). **(C)** Axial T1-weighted image (WI) shows low T1 signal (*arrows*) in some of the lesions. **(D)** Axial T1WI after gadolinium administration shows peripheral (*arrowhead*) and central (*arrow*) enhancement in some of the lesions.

## ■ Differential Diagnosis

- *Multiple sclerosis (MS):* Characteristic MS lesions are periventricular in location and ovoid in shape, and they may or may not show enhancement, which is often ringlike. Lesions in the corpus callosum, the brainstem beyond the pons, and the spinal cord increase the specificity for MS.
- *Chronic small-vessel ischemic disease:* This is characterized by T2 hyperintensities in the white matter, which are frequently seen in patients of advanced age. The usual location is in the periventricular and subcortical white matter. Infratentorial lesions may present in the pons, but rarely elsewhere.
- *Vasculitis:* Vasculitis causes neurologic dysfunction and multiple focal ischemic lesions in persons of the same age range as those prone to MS. Abnormalities of the corpus callosum, optic nerves, and spinal cord may allow MS to be differentiated from vascular disease.

## ■ Essential Facts

- MS is an autoimmune inflammatory neurologic disease characterized by demyelination and axonal injury.
- MS presents as multiple lesions that are more periventricular than peripheral and have an ovoid shape; at the initial stage, the lesions are typically thin and appear to be linear (Dawson fingers). Other characteristics include dilated perivascular spaces; lesions in the subcortical region, brainstem, U-fibers, optic nerves, corpus callosum, and visual pathway; and generalized atrophy at a relatively young age.
- MS generally presents in young adults. A female predominance is noted. Clinical features include optic neuritis, transverse myelitis, internuclear ophthalmoplegia, and paresthesias or variable signs of neuropsychological dysfunction.

## ■ Other Imaging Findings

- Conventional magnetic resonance imaging (MRI) findings:
  - Lesions are bright on T2WIs and FLAIR images.
  - On T1WIs, acute MS lesions are isointense to normal white matter and hypointense if chronic tissue injury or severe inflammatory edema has occurred; the accumulation of hypointense lesions (so-called black holes) may correlate with progression of disease and disability.
- The lesions enhance in the acute inflammatory phase and may vary in shape and size. They usually start as homogeneous enhancing nodules. Subsequent progression to ringlike enhancement is noted.
- Magnetization transfer imaging can detect areas of normal-appearing white matter with abnormal magnetization transfer ratios arising from myelin loss. It may also help to differentiate MS plaques from small-vessel ischemic disease.

## ✓ Pearls & ✗ Pitfalls

- ✓ The ability to detect MS lesions with MRI increases with the field strength.
- ✓ The number and size of enhancing lesions detected on MRI can be increased with the use of a triple dose or three sequential single doses of gadolinium. Enhancement is suggestive of new lesion formation and inflammatory activity.
- ✓ Numerous cortical lesions have been observed on histopathologic examination, but they are not commonly seen on conventional MRI.
- ✗ FLAIR images are usually optimized for contrast between lesions, white matter, and gray matter, and they may be less sensitive in detecting brainstem lesions. Proton-density WIs and T2WIs are more reliable for the detection of lesions in this location.

# Case 86

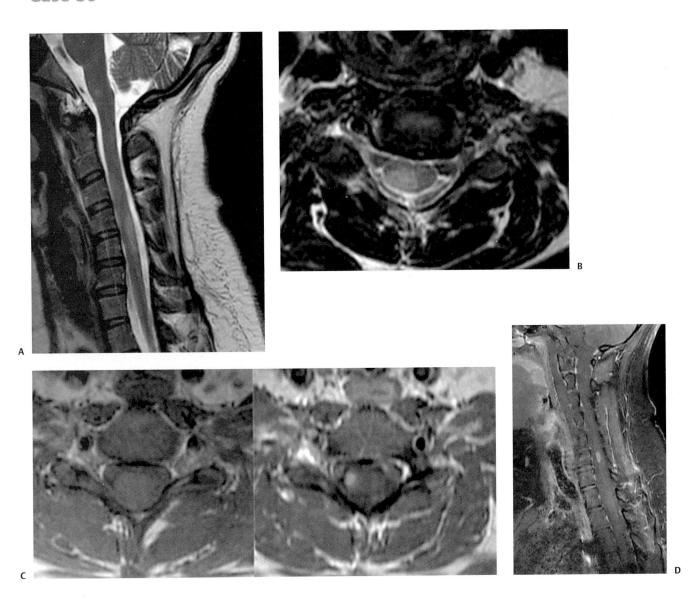

## Clinical Presentation

A 42-year-old woman with paresthesias in both arms.

## ■ Imaging Findings

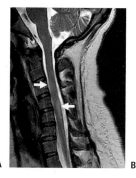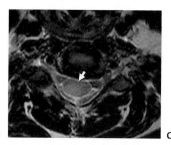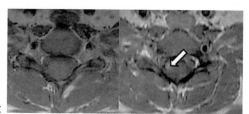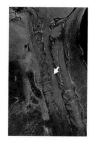

(A) Sagittal T2-weighted image (WI) of the cord shows multiple oval areas of increased signal in the ventral and dorsal cord spanning the length of one to two vertebral bodies (*arrows*). (B) Axial T2WI of the cervical spine shows a wedge-shaped peripheral cord lesion dorsally (*arrow*). (C) Axial T1WI before and after gadolinium injection. Note the enhancement of one of the cord lesions (*arrow*). (D) Sagittal fat-suppressed T1WI shows a cigar-shaped enhancing cord lesion that spans less than the height of one vertebral body (*arrow*).

## ■ Differential Diagnosis

• **Multiple sclerosis (MS) in the cord:** This is characterized by peripherally located focal cord lesions that are less than two vertebral segments in length and occupy less than half of the cross-sectional area of the cord. In the axial images, the lesions may have a wedge shape, with the base at the cord surface, or a round shape if there is no contact with the cord surface.

• *Devic neuromyelitis optica:* This is a demyelinating disease characterized by bilateral visual disturbance and transverse myelopathy. It may have a mono- or multiphasic course. Longitudinal, confluent lesions extending across five or more vertebral segments with hyperintensity on T2WIs are common. Cord swelling and enhancement may be present.

• *Transverse myelitis (TM):* TM is a clinical syndrome characterized by bilateral motor, sensory, and autonomic disturbances. There is perivascular monocytic and lymphocytic infiltration, demyelination, and axonal injury. TM may be part of a multifocal central nervous system disease, a multisystemic disease, or an isolated, idiopathic entity. The lesions are centrally located and hyperintense, and they usually occupy more than two-thirds of the cross-sectional area of the cord and have a length of more than three to four vertebral segments. Cord expansion may or may not be present. Enhancement is infrequent. TM may be patchy or diffuse.

## ■ Essential Facts

• MS is a chronic inflammatory demyelinating disease of the central nervous system that can lead to irreversible tissue loss or partial demyelination.

• The spinal cord is frequently involved in MS, either alone or with the brain.

• As many as 25% of cases have been found to involve only the spinal cord.

• The clinical presentation includes motor, sensory, or sphincter dysfunction.

• Most spinal cord lesions occur in the cervical region.

• Cord swelling is usually found only in the relapsing-remitting form of MS.

• The incidence of enhancing lesions in the spine is significantly lower than the incidence in the brain.

• Cord atrophy can be due to inflammatory tissue injury, demyelination, and axonal loss.

## ■ Other Imaging Findings

• On magnetic resonance imaging (MRI), demyelinating plaques are hyperintense on T2WIs.

• In the spine, on sagittal sections, plaques have a cigar shape and may be located centrally, anteriorly, or dorsally. Diffuse lesions are seen as mild intramedullary hyperintensities on T2WIs.

• In the brain, lesions are seen as multiple white matter lesions in the pericallosal region, brainstem, optic nerves, corpus callosum, and visual pathways.

• Chronic lesions are hypointense on T1WIs.

• Lesions, which may vary in shape and size, enhance in the acute inflammatory phase. The enhancement starts as homogeneous nodules and subsequently progresses to ringlike enhancing lesions.

## ✓ Pearls & ✗ Pitfalls

✓ Chronic foci of hypointensity on T1WIs of the brain, known as black holes, are not present in the spinal cord.

✗ Spinal cord imaging is prone to multiple artifacts:

   • Motion: subject motion, blood flow, respiratory motion, swallowing, cerebrospinal fluid pulsation

   • Susceptibility artifacts: interfaces (bone and soft tissue, fat and air), trabecular bone, metallic implants

   • Chemical shift artifacts: epidural and vertebral fat

# Case 87

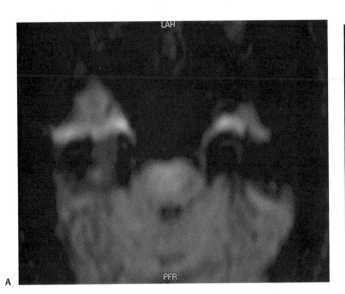

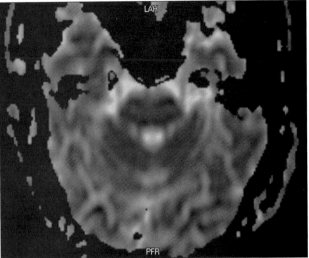

## Clinical Presentation

A 68-year-old with the recent onset of spastic quadriparesis.

## Further Work-up

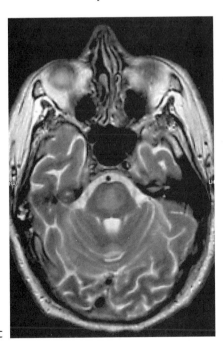

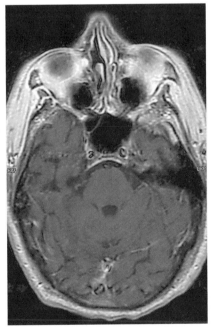

■ **Imaging Findings**

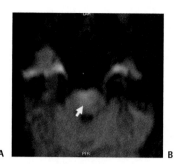
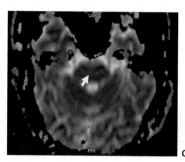
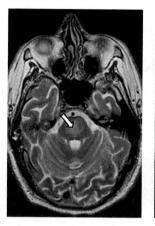
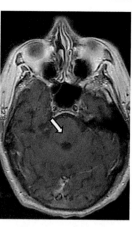

**(A)** Diffusion-weighted image (WI) shows an area of increased signal without corresponding low signal on the apparent diffusion coefficient (ADC) map, consistent with T2 shine-through (*arrow*). **(B)** ADC map does not show decreased signal in the area of diffusion abnormality, indicating T2 shine-through (*arrow*). **(C)** Axial T2WI demonstrates an area of high signal in the central portion of the pons (*arrow*). **(D)** Axial T1WI after gadolinium contrast fails to demonstrate enhancement or T1 signal change.

■ **Differential Diagnosis**

• ***Central pontine myelinolysis (CPM):*** CPM is an osmolar disturbance resulting in demyelination and is part of the osmotic demyelination syndrome. Acute demyelination in the pons results in symmetric areas of signal abnormality in the central pons on T2WIs. The appearance on diffusion-WIs is variable. No contrast enhancement is present.

• *Posterior reversible encephalopathy syndrome:* This is the result of neurotoxicity-induced vasogenic edema. It more frequently involves the cerebral hemispheres but may present with lesions in the basal ganglia, brainstem, and deep white matter (external/internal capsule).

• *Acute pontine infarct:* Patients present with the sudden onset of neurologic deficit. There is restricted diffusion preceding a T2 signal increase. Vertebral or basilar occlusive changes may or may not be present.

■ **Essential Facts**

• Patients who are chronic alcoholics, malnourished, transplant recipients, or chronically debilitated are at risk.

• CPM is associated with electrolyte abnormalities, including hyponatremia, which is rapidly overcorrected.

• Extrapontine myelinolysis occurs in the white matter of the cerebellum, thalamus, globus pallidus, putamen, and lateral geniculate body.

• The clinical course is biphasic; generalized encephalopathy is caused by the hyponatremia, which usually improves transiently following an initial elevation of the sodium level.

• Spastic quadriparesis and pseudobulbar palsy develop 2 to 3 days later as a consequence of myelinolysis.

■ **Other Imaging Findings**

• Magnetic resonance imaging (MRI):
  • Symmetric areas of signal intensity abnormality in the central pons are seen on T2WIs and fluid-attenuated inversion recovery images. The corticospinal tracts are spared.
  • The condition may progress to classic hyperintense "trident-shaped" CPM, with sparing of the ventrolateral pons and corticospinal tracts.
  • Restricted diffusion may be seen before the T2 signal abnormalities.

✓ **Pearls & ✗ Pitfalls**

✓ The diagnosis of CPM is not ruled out in the setting of normal imaging findings.

✓ MRI changes may be delayed.

✓ The severity of the MRI findings is not prognostic.

✗ In the absence of a clinical history of sodium shifts, asymptomatic pontine lesions are unlikely to be CPM lesions.

*Case courtesy of Alexander Simonetta, MD.*

# Case 88

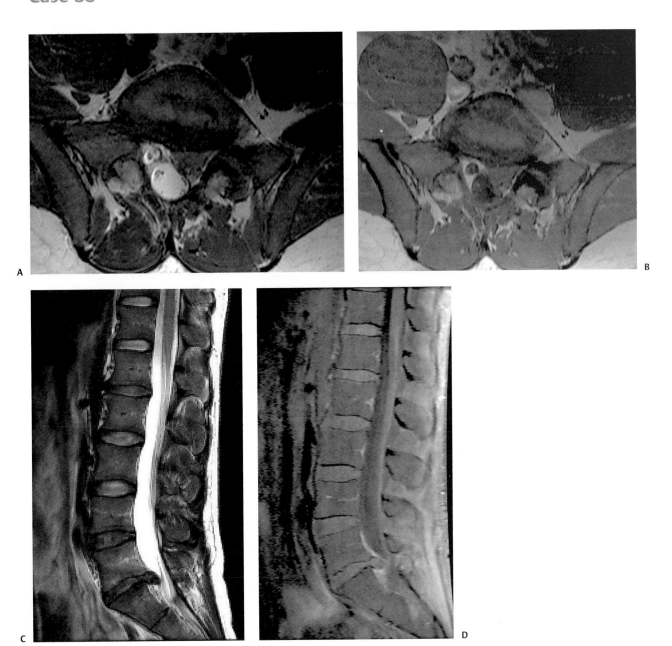

A

B

C

D

## Clinical Presentation

A 52-year-old with numbness in the left foot.

### ◾ Imaging Findings

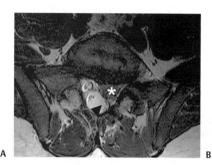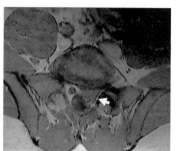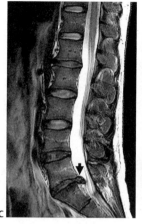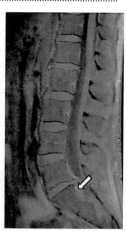

**(A)** Axial T2-weighted image (WI) at the level of the L5-S1 intervertebral disk shows an oval mass continuous with the disk occupying the left lateral recess (*asterisk*). Note the posterior displacement of the left S1 nerve root (*arrowhead*). **(B)** Axial T1WI at the level of the L5-S1 intervertebral disk. Note the thin plane of fat that separates the lesion from the facet joint (*arrow*). **(C)** Observe the continuity of the lesion with the L5-S1 disk on the sagittal T2WI (*arrow*). **(D)** Sagittal fat-suppressed T1WI shows enhancement of the epidural plexus (*arrow*), but not of the disk herniation.

### ◾ Differential Diagnosis

- **Disk herniation:** This is a localized displacement of disk material beyond the limits of the intervertebral disk space. It encroaches on the epidural fat and sometimes the dural sac and nerve roots. The herniation is usually contiguous with the rest of the disk, but free fragments are possible. The herniation is usually isointense to the parent disk on T1- and T2-weighted sequences.
- *Facet synovial cyst:* This frequently occupies the lateral recess and may extend to the central canal. Cysts can contain synovial serous fluid, more gelatinous material, air, or blood. They are continuous with the facet joint but may abut the disk as well.
- *Epidural hematoma:* This is an epidural collection with variable signal intensity depending on the blood products contained therein. Epidural hematoma may span more than one level.

### ◾ Essential Facts

- Degenerative disk disease is more common in the elderly population; however, acute herniations are frequent in the middle-aged population.
- Disk herniation is defined as the localized displacement of disk material beyond the normal margins of the intervertebral disk space.
  - Protrusion: the greatest distance, in any plane, between the edges of the disk material beyond the disk space is less than the distance between the edges of the base in the same plane.
  - Extrusion: any one distance between the edges of the disk material beyond the disk space is greater than the distance between the edges of the base in the same plane.

- When there is no contiguity with the parent disk, the extruded material may be characterized as a sequestered or free fragment.
- Relative to the axial plane, the herniation may be central, right or left central, right or left subarticular, right or left foraminal, or right or left extraforaminal.

### ◾ Other Imaging Findings

- Magnetic resonance imaging (MRI) is the technique most frequently used for the evaluation of disk herniation.
- Computed tomography is more accurate than MRI for the identification of calcified herniations and associated bony abnormalities, such as posterior accompanying osteophytes.
- In provocation lumbar diskography, direct disk stimulation is used to help identify the specific disk(s) responsible for lower back pain.

### ✓ Pearls & ✗ Pitfalls

✓ MRI can be used to follow nontreated disk herniations.

✓ The main MRI findings useful to presume spontaneous regression of disk herniations after 6 months are free fragments, T2-weighted hyperintense herniation, peripheral enhancement after gadolinium administration, and recent clinical onset.

✗ After gadolinium injection, many herniations show a thin enhancing rim that is caused by the inflammatory reaction.

✗ A contrast agent is more widely used in postoperative examinations because it is useful for differentiating residual or recurrent herniations from scar tissue.

# Case 89

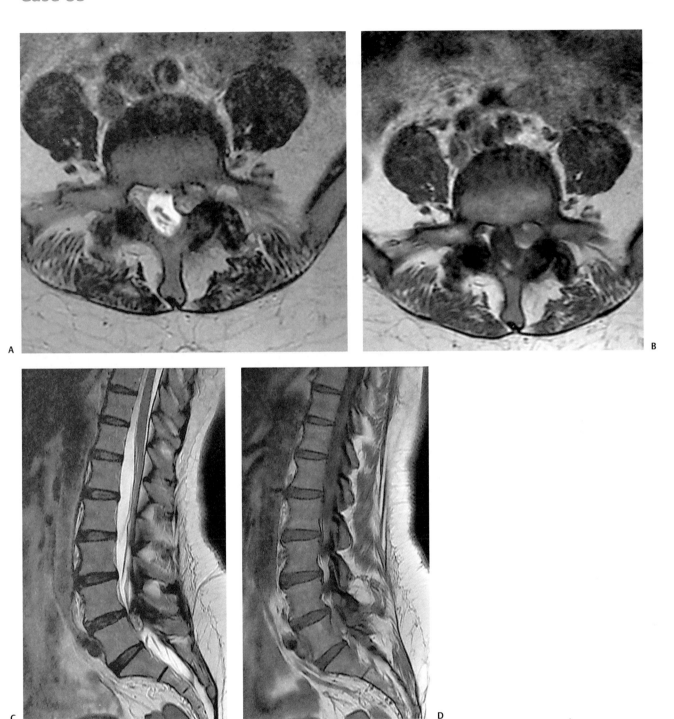

## Clinical Presentation

A 46-year-old with weakness and pain in the left leg.

### ■ Imaging Findings

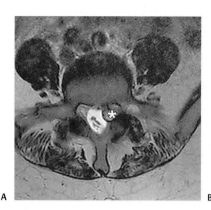
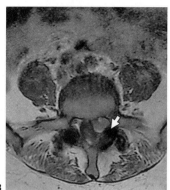
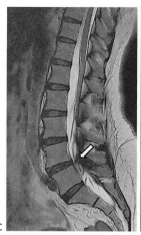
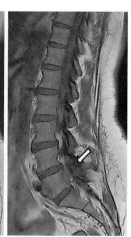

A    B    C    D

**(A)** Axial T1-weighted image (WI) at the level of L4-L5 demonstrates an oval lesion in the left lateral recess with a rim of low signal and central heterogeneous high signal (*asterisk*). The left L5 nerve root cannot be separated from the mass. **(B)** Axial T1WI shows heterogeneous high signal in the left lateral recess lesion, which abuts the facet joint (*arrow*). **(C)** Sagittal T2WI shows the close relationship of the lesion with the facet joint (*arrow*). There is no contact with the intervertebral disk. **(D)** Sagittal T1WI shows the close relationship of the lesion with the facet joint (*arrow*). There is no contact with the intervertebral disk.

### ■ Differential Diagnosis

- ***Facet synovial cyst:*** Facet synovial cysts frequently occupy the lateral recess and may extend to central spinal canal. Cysts can contain synovial serous fluid, more gelatinous material, air, or blood. They are continuous with the facet joint but may abut the disk as well.
- *Disk herniation:* This causes a focal contour abnormality along the posterior disk margin that displaces the epidural fat and sometimes the dural sac and nerve roots. The herniation is usually contiguous with the rest of the disk, but free fragments are possible.
- *Meningioma:* This is usually an intradural extramedullary mass. It appears isointense to the spinal cord on both T1WIs and T2WIs but may be hypointense on T1WIs and hyperintense on T2WIs. Homogeneous intense enhancement is present.

### ■ Essential Facts

- Facet joints are frequently involved in spondyloarthrosis.
- The typical imaging findings are joint space narrowing, subchondral sclerosis, cysts, osteophytosis, ligament thickening, intra-articular vacuum, and joint fluid.
- Severe facet osteoarthritis can cause lateral recess and neural foramen stenosis.
- Facet joint degeneration is complicated by synovial cysts, which originate from the joint and can keep or lose their connection with the joint.

### ■ Other Imaging Findings

- Plain films can show degenerative changes; however, the anatomic complexity of this region requires computed tomography (CT) or magnetic resonance imaging (MRI) for a complete evaluation of the degenerative process.
- CT is more accurate for identifying bony abnormalities, but MRI more clearly shows the neural structures and soft tissues.

### ✓ Pearls & ✗ Pitfalls

- ✓ The role of facet joints in back pain is often difficult to assess because the symptoms can be unspecific and imaging findings of degeneration are common.
- ✓ In selected cases, nerve block or steroid and anesthetic injections of the facet joint are useful for diagnostic and therapeutic purposes.
- ✗ Spondylolysis may result in heterogeneous signal in the vicinity of the facets and should not be mistaken for synovial cyst formation.

# Case 90

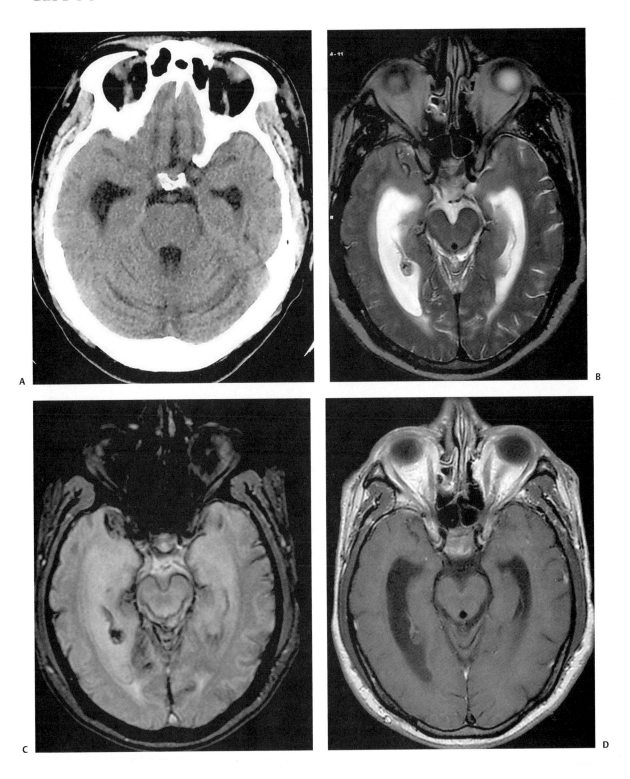

## ▪ Clinical Presentation

A 57-year-old man with three prior episodes of intraventricular hemorrhage and secondary hydrocephalus, now presenting with bilateral hearing loss and ataxia.

### ■ Imaging Findings

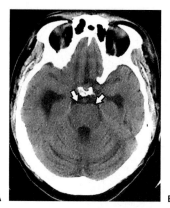
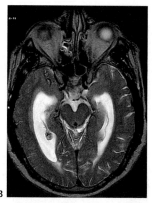
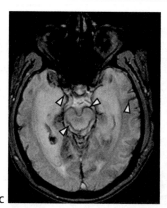
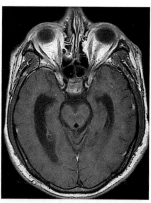

A    B    C    D

**(A)** Axial computed tomography without contrast shows a thin rim of high intensity on the anterior aspect of the pons (*arrows*). There is cerebellar atrophy with prominence of the sulci and hydrocephalus. **(B)** Axial fast spin-echo (FSE) T2-weighted image (WI) shows a rim of low intensity on the surface of the central nervous system. **(C)** Axial gradient-echo (GRE) T2*WI of the brain shows a thick rim of dark signal on the surface of the central nervous system (*arrowheads*). **(D)** Axial T1WI with contrast shows no abnormal enhancement.

### ■ Differential Diagnosis

- **Superficial siderosis:** Deposits of hemosiderin on the surface of the central nervous system (CNS) occur in some patients after multiple episodes of intraventricular or subarachnoid hemorrhage. A rim of low intensity in the surface of the CNS is best seen on GRE T2*WIs. There is no enhancement.
- *Leptomeningeal melanin:* An increased amount of melanin in the leptomeninges can be an anatomic variant. It is seen as a thick, T2-hypointense rim on the surface of the medulla oblongata. GRE T2*WIs do not show these findings. Evaluation of the degree of skin pigmentation (individuals with heavier skin pigmentation demonstrate denser leptomeningeal pigmentation) and the absence of any other pathologic leptomeningeal characteristics may aid in the differentiation of this entity from iron- or melanin-containing diffuse leptomeningeal diseases.
- *Magnetic resonance artifacts:* T1 or T2 shortening of the brain surface is seen as a rim of hypointensity of variable thickness on the surface of the brain. This is evidenced only in certain sequences.

### ■ Essential Facts

- Superficial siderosis is an uncommon condition.
- Reactive gliosis and demyelination affect the cerebellum and cranial nerves I through VIII.
- A minimal rim of increased density will be present on the CNS surface, with cerebral and cerebellar atrophy.

### ■ Other Imaging Findings

- GRE T2*WIs show a hemosiderin rim on the surface of the CNS because of the susceptibility artifact of hemosiderin.
- FSE T2WIs show a dark rim on the CNS surface.
- Typically, no enhancement is seen.

### ✓ Pearls & ✗ Pitfalls

- ✓ Many times, superficial siderosis is an incidental finding, manifesting only if gliosis is present.
- ✓ A history of repeated intracranial hemorrhage is the usual scenario.
- ✗ Always ask for GRE T2*WIs if superficial siderosis is suspected because the sensitivity of the other imaging sequences for detecting this entity is poor.
- ✗ In half of cases, the cause of siderosis is not identified.

# Case 91

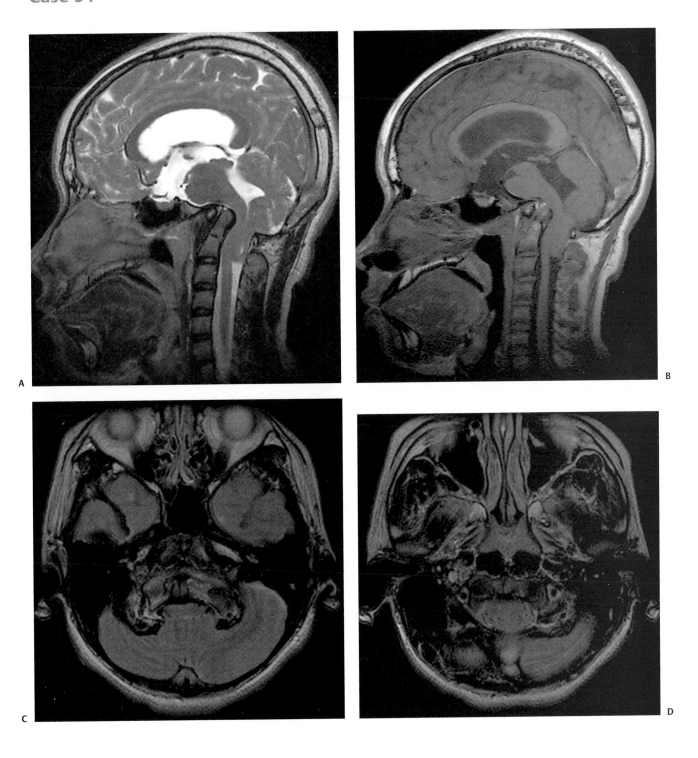

A

B

C

D

## Clinical Presentation

A 17-year-old with a history of hydrocephalus.

### ■ Imaging Findings

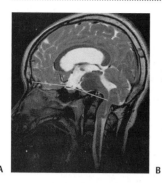
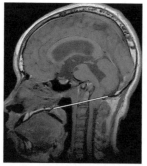
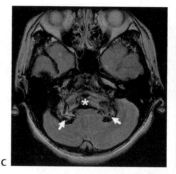
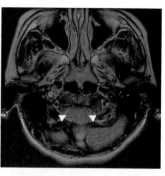

**(A)** Sagittal T2-weighted image (WI) of the brain: The basal angle measures 176 degrees. This angle is subtended by the junction of the nasion-tuberculum and tuberculum-basion tangents. Average is 134 to 135 degrees, minimum is 121 degrees, and maximum is 148 to 149 degrees. Consider platybasia if the angle is greater than 150 degrees. **(B)** Sagittal T1WI of the brain: The Chamberlain line extends from the posterior margin of the hard palate to the opisthion (posterior margin of the foramen magnum). It is abnormal if the tip of the odontoid projects more than 5 mm above the Chamberlain line. **(C)** Axial T2WI at the level of the foramen magnum demonstrates the tip of the dens (*asterisk*) at the same level as the occipital condyles (*arrows*). Note the compressive effect on the medulla oblongata. **(D)** Axial T2WI again demonstrates the compressive effect on the medulla oblongata and on the cerebellar tonsils (*arrowheads*), which are low-lying.

### ■ Differential Diagnosis

- **Basilar invagination and platybasia:** This is a developmental abnormality in which the vertebral column is situated in an abnormally high position because of decreased height of the skull base. The odontoid tip lies more than 5 mm above the Chamberlain line (posterior margin of hard palate to opisthion); the anterior arch of C1 typically lies below. The tip of the odontoid is located more than 7 mm above the McGregor line (posterior margin of hard palate to the lowest point of the occipital squamosal surface); the anterior arch of C1 typically lies below. The base of the skull is congenitally flat.
- *Chiari type I malformation:* This is characterized by a caudal extension of the cerebellar tonsils below the foramen magnum. It may present in isolation or be associated with shortening of the clivus, basilar invagination, C1 assimilation, and fused cervical vertebrae (Klipper-Feil syndrome).
- *Sagging brain:* This is secondary to spinal hypotension and may present spontaneously or after spinal procedures; it may also be due to cerebrospinal fluid leak. The brainstem and 3rd ventricle "sag" inferiorly, and the pituitary gland is upwardly convex. If contrast is administered, dural thickening and enhancement are demonstrated.

### ■ Essential Facts

- *Basilar impression* refers to the acquired form of basilar invagination, associated with conditions that soften the skull base, such as osteogenesis imperfecta, hyperparathyroidism, rickets, and Paget disease.
- *Platybasia* refers to flattening of the skull base. It may be present in patients with basilar invagination and basilar impression, but these conditions may exist in the absence of platybasia.

- Other abnormalities of the craniovertebral junction may coexist:
  - Basiocciput hypoplasia (short clivus)
  - Occipital condyle hypoplasia
  - Atlanto-occipital nonsegmentation (i.e., assimilation or occipitalization of the atlas)
  - Atlas anomalies
  - Axis anomalies (os odontoideum, aplasia, or hypoplasia of the dens)

### ■ Other Imaging Findings

- Plain radiographs are inaccurate for measurements because of the superimposition of osseous structures.
- Computed tomography provides optimal visualization of the osseous structures.
- Magnetic resonance imaging (MRI) also permits assessment of the surrounding soft-tissue structures and cervicomedullary junction.

### ✓ Pearls & ✗ Pitfalls

- ✓ Numerous syndromes may involve the craniovertebral junction and cause atlantoaxial instability:
  - Klippel-Feil syndrome
  - Down syndrome
  - Connective tissue disorders, such as Ehlers-Danlos syndrome
  - Inflammatory conditions such as rheumatoid arthritis and oropharyngeal infections
  - Achondroplasia
  - Mucopolysaccharidoses
  - Osteogenesis imperfecta
- ✗ In the assessment for platybasia, measurement of the basal angles with MRI yields lower values than those previously reported with traditional radiography.

# Case 92

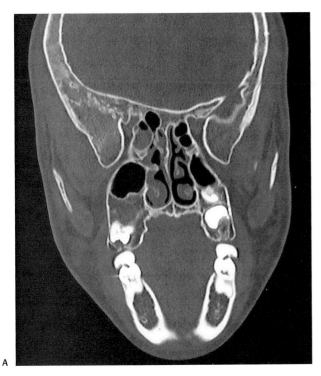
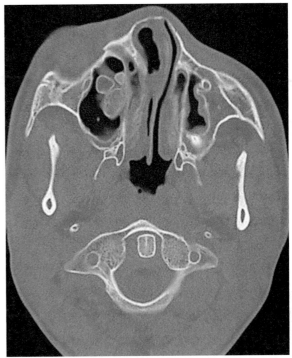

## Clinical Presentation

A 36-year-old woman with long-standing cosmetic deformity of the face.

## Further Work-up

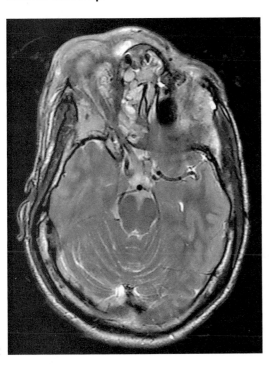
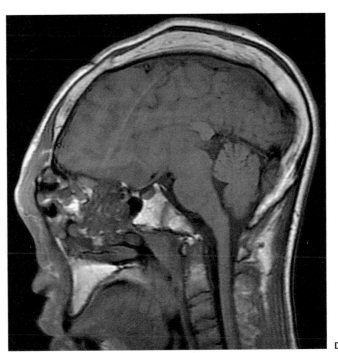

## ■ Imaging Findings

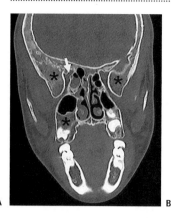
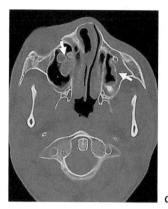
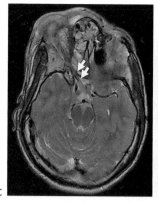
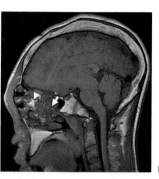

A   B   C   D

**(A)** Reformatted coronal computed tomography (CT) of the face shows replacement and enlargement of the bone marrow in the greater sphenoid wing and maxillary bones (*asterisks*), predominantly on the right, with a ground glass attenuation. Note the narrowing of the right superior orbital fissure (*arrow*) in comparison with the left. **(B)** Axial CT shows proliferation of abnormal bone marrow within the right maxillary sinus and lateral wall of the left maxillary sinus (*arrows*). Asymmetry of the face is evident. **(C)** Axial T2-weighted image (WI) through the orbital roof shows heterogeneous signal of the abnormal bone marrow. Note the elongation of the right optic nerve (*arrows*) and proptosis, caused by the enlarged orbital walls. **(D)** Sagittal T1WI shows that the areas of marrow replacement display relatively low signal (*arrow*). Areas of high T1 signal within the ethmoid complex may represent secretions or secondary retention of mucus (*arrowhead*). Note the magnetic susceptibility artifact in the region of the nasion, secondary to prior surgery.

## ■ Differential Diagnosis

- *Fibrous dysplasia (FD):* FD presents with deformity of the face secondary to enlargement of multiple bones and abnormal attenuation of the bone. The skull base foramina may be distorted.
- *Paget disease (PD):* PD is a chronic progressive disease of unknown etiology in which initial destruction of bone is followed by a reparative process. The radiographic changes are progressive and include osteoporosis circumscripta, enlargement of the skull, thickening of the outer table, and finally complete sclerosis with loss of distinction between the diploë and calvarial bone tables.
- *Chronic invasive fungal sinusitis:* Inhaled fungal organisms invade the mucosa, submucosa, blood vessels, and bony walls of the paranasal sinuses. On CT, a hyperattenuating soft-tissue collection within one or more of the paranasal sinuses is present. It may be masslike, with destruction of the sinus walls and extension beyond the confines of the sinus. On magnetic resonance imaging (MRI), there may be decreased signal intensity on T1WIs and markedly decreased signal intensity on T2WIs.

## ■ Essential Facts

- FD is a benign bone condition of unknown etiology in which normal bone is replaced by an abnormal proliferation of fibroconnective tissue.
- The three types are monostotic, polyostotic, and polyostotic with cutaneous and endocrine abnormalities (McCune-Albright syndrome).
- Craniofacial FD may affect the base of the skull, orbits, maxillae, and mandibles; symptoms result from the mass effect exerted by the lesion; cranial neuropathies may result from involvement of the foramina.

- The radiographic appearance includes intramedullary lesions that distort and expand the bone, mixed radiolucent and radiopaque lesions, "ground-glass" attenuation, and narrowing of the skull base foramina.

## ■ Other Imaging Findings

- CT shows patterns similar to those visible on plain radiography and assesses the compromise of the skull base foramina.
- MRI shows variable signal intensity, usually intermediate signal on T1WIs and hypointense signal on T2WIs.
- Scintigraphy demonstrates increased uptake of the radioisotope. It may be useful for the detection of subtle pathologic fractures.

## ✓ Pearls & ✗ Pitfalls

✓ Tips to differentiate FD from PD:
  - "Ground-glass" bone matrix is typical of FD but is not seen in PD.
  - FD tends to affect cranial bones asymmetrically, whereas the cranium is symmetric in PD.
  - The paranasal sinuses are not usually involved in PD.
  - The cortical tables are thick in PD (especially the inner table) but tend to be thin in FD.

✗ Sites of high signal intensity on T2WIs in the frontoethmoid area should raise the possibility of a coexistent mucocele.

# Case 93

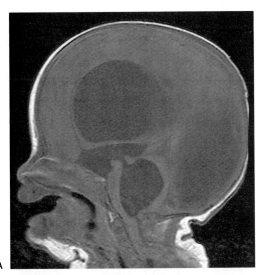

A

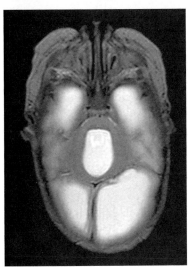

B

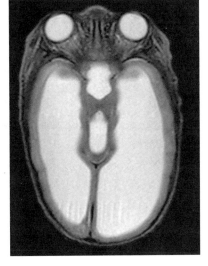

C

## ■ Clinical Presentation

A 30-week premature infant, now 3 months of age, presenting with increased head circumference.

## Further Work-up

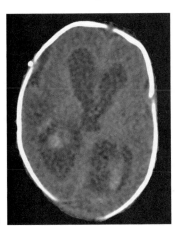

D

### ■ Imaging Findings

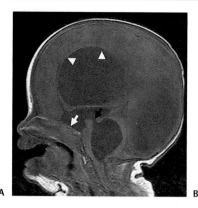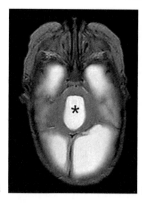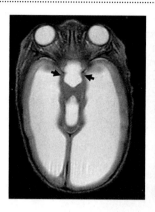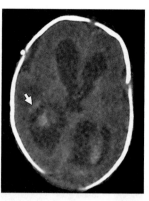

A   B   C   D

**(A)** Sagittal T1-weighted image (WI) shows dilatation of the entire ventricular system. Note the elongation and thinning of the corpus callosum (*arrowheads*), descent of the floor of the 3rd ventricle, which is obliterating the suprasellar cistern and abutting the pituitary gland (*white arrow*), and enlargement of the aqueduct (*black arrow*) and 4th ventricle. **(B)** Axial T2WI shows that the anteroposterior diameter of the 4th ventricle (*asterisk*) is significantly increased, resulting in flattening of the dorsal surface of the pons. **(C)** Axial T2WI shows that the dilated 3rd ventricle occupies the suprasellar cistern. The hypothalamic structures are splayed (*arrows*). **(D)** Computed tomography of the brain obtained 3 months earlier, when the patient was 2 weeks old. Intraventricular hemorrhage and mild ventricular dilatation are evident. Note the parenchymal hemorrhage in the right periventricular white matter (*arrow*).

### ■ Differential Diagnosis

- **Communicating hydrocephalus:** Enlargement of the ventricular system and obliteration of the extra-axial spaces. There may be a history of prior intraventricular hemorrhage or meningitis.
- *Hydranencephaly:* The cerebral hemispheres are replaced by cerebrospinal fluid (CSF), with preservation of the thalami, inferior aspect of the frontal lobes, and inferior and medial aspect of the temporal lobes. Atrophy of the brainstem may be present. The cerebellum is usually normal. The key to distinguishing hydrocephalus from hydranencephaly is the presence of a thin rim of residual cerebral cortical tissue in hydrocephalus that is not present in hydranencephaly. Vascular, infectious, and genetic causes have been implicated.
- *Severe brain atrophy:* Enlargement of the ventricular system and prominent extra-axial spaces, secondary to loss of brain volume, are characteristic. Elongation of the corpus callosum, descent of the 3rd ventricular floor, ballooning of the 3rd ventricle, and lateral displacement of the hypothalamic structures are indicative of increased pressure within the ventricles and are absent in passive ventricular enlargement.

### ■ Essential Facts

- Hydrocephalus is defined as ventricular dilatation and increased pressure resulting from an imbalance between CSF production and absorption.
- It is associated with the following:
  - Ventricular enlargement
  - Effacement of the extra-axial spaces
  - Dilatation of the 3rd ventricle, downward displacement of 3rd ventricular floor, and splaying of the hypothalamic nuclei

- Transependymal flow of CSF
- Communicating hydrocephalus:
  - The CSF flow blockage is outside the ventricular system (e.g., basal cisterns or parasagittal arachnoid villi).
  - Causes include meningitis, subarachnoid hemorrhage, meningeal carcinomatosis, and abnormal skull base.
- Noncommunicating hydrocephalus:
  - There is intraventricular obstruction (at or proximal to the 4th ventricular outlets).
  - The dilatation of the segments of the ventricular system is proximal to the obstruction.

### ■ Other Imaging Findings

- CSF flow voids are accentuated on magnetic resonance imaging (MRI).
- Signal abnormalities can be found within the corpus callosum after ventricular shunting and are probably caused by compression of the corpus callosum against the falx before ventricular decompression.

### ✓ Pearls & ✗ Pitfalls

- ✓ Rapid-sequence MRI has been used for the nonemergent imaging evaluation of pediatric hydrocephalus.
- ✓ MRI yields reliable visualization of the ventricular catheter and offers superior anatomic detail while limiting exposure to radiation.
- ✗ Periventricular edema due to transependymal CSF flow or hydrostatic stasis from elevated intraventricular pressure may be evident as blurred or ill-defined ventricular margins. This finding favors acute or subacute or progressive hydrocephalus; however, in an infant, the normally high water content of the immature white matter may obscure the edema.

# Case 94

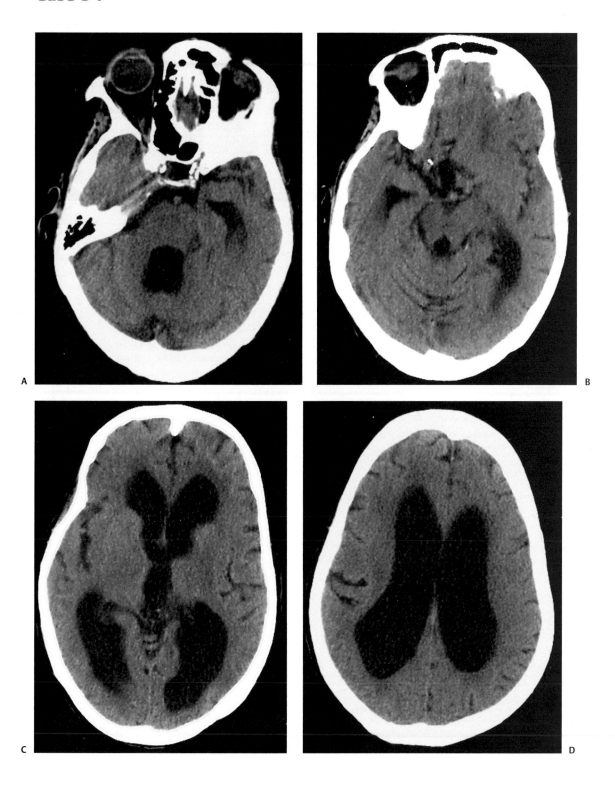

## Clinical Presentation

A 72-year-old with gait disturbance and memory loss.

■ **Imaging Findings**

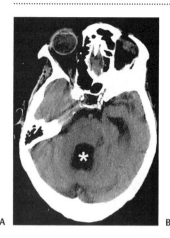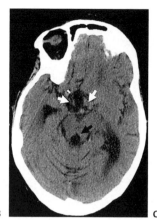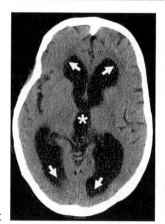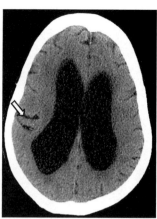

(A) Axial computed tomography (CT) at the level of the pons shows dilatation of the 4th ventricle (*asterisk*). Note the prominence of the left temporal horn. (B) At the level of the midbrain, a large aqueduct (*black arrow*) and splaying of the hypothalamic structures (*white arrows*) are demonstrated. (C) There is fusiform dilatation of the 3rd ventricle (*asterisk*) and a round configuration of the frontal and occipital horns (*white arrows*). Note the small size of the sylvian fissures relative to the enlarged ventricles. (D) At the level of the corona radiata, there is only minimal sulcal enlargement (*arrow*).

■ **Differential Diagnosis**

- **Normal-pressure hydrocephalus (NPH):** This is one of the few treatable causes of dementia. There is dilatation of the entire ventricular system without commensurate sulcal dilatation.
- *Diffuse cerebral atrophy:* This is associated with volume loss of the cortex and white matter, resulting in enlargement of the ventricles and sulci. The 3rd ventricle is usually not dilated, and there is no splaying of the hypothalamic structures.
- *Obstructive hydrocephalus:* This is indicated by dilatation of the ventricular system above the level of an intra- or extraventricular lesion. The obstruction is proximal to the 4th ventricular outlets.

■ **Essential Facts**

- Clinical findings of NPH include gait difficulty, cognitive decline, incontinence of urine, and enlarged ventricles.
- Hydrocephalus is not secondary to such conditions as head trauma, intracerebral hemorrhage, and meningitis.
- CT and magnetic resonance imaging show ventriculomegaly with minimal or no sulcal enlargement and minimal or absent periventricular increased signal on T2-weighted images, indicating a chronic process.

✓ **Pearls & ✗ Pitfalls**

✓ Since it was first described, the definition of NPH has been expanded. Initially, it was considered to be idiopathic; at present, any form of chronic communicating hydrocephalus and even a few noncommunicating forms, such as aqueductal stenosis, are included.

✗ All the cardinal features of NPH (gait difficulty, cognitive decline, incontinence of urine, and enlarged ventricles) are common in the elderly and have many causes.

# Case 95

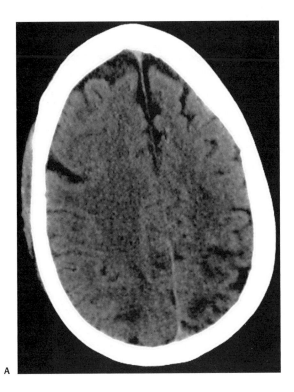

A

## Clinical Presentation

A patient who has a history of lung cancer treated with chemotherapy now presents with headache and altered mentation.

## Further Work-up

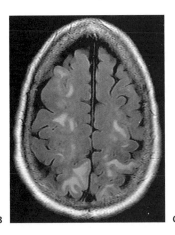

B

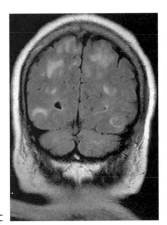

C

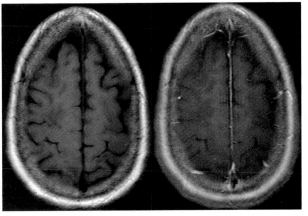

D

### ■ Imaging Findings

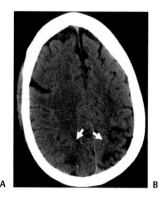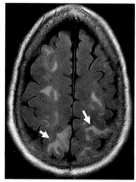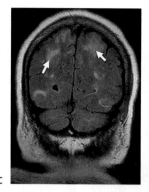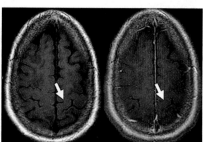

**(A)** Axial computed tomography (CT) of the brain shows areas of low attenuation in the subcortical white matter of both parietal lobes, without mass effect (*arrows*). **(B)** Axial fluid-attenuated inversion recovery (FLAIR) image demonstrates vasogenic edema in the frontal and parietal subcortical white matter bilaterally (*arrows*). **(C)** Coronal FLAIR image demonstrates vasogenic edema in the frontal and parietal subcortical white matter bilaterally (*arrows*). **(D)** Axial T1-weighted images (WIs) before and after gadolinium injection fail to demonstrate contrast enhancement (*arrows*).

### ■ Differential Diagnosis

- ***Posterior reversible encephalopathy syndrome (PRES):*** Vasogenic edema is seen in the subcortical white mater of both parietal and occipital regions. There is no abnormal enhancement or significant mass effect.
- *Watershed cerebral infarctions:* Cytotoxic edema would be evident on the diffusion-WIs. Watershed infarcts involve the deep white matter in a "rosary of pearls" pattern, or the cortex at the junction of the anterior and middle cerebral artery territories or the middle and posterior cerebral artery territories.
- *Brain metastasis:* Vasogenic edema is caused by multiple focal enhancing lesions. There is no predilection for watershed zones.

### ■ Essential Facts

- PRES is the result of neurotoxicity-induced vasogenic edema.
- Associated conditions:
  - Toxemia of pregnancy (preeclampsia/eclampsia)
  - After transplant
  - Immunosuppression (cyclosporine, tacrolimus)
  - Infection, sepsis, shock
  - Autoimmune diseases
  - After cancer chemotherapy
  - Other conditions: dialysis/erythropoietin, triple-H (hypertensive, hypervolemic, hemodilution) therapy
- On CT/magnetic resonance (MR) imaging, the brain typically demonstrates symmetric focal regions of hemispheric edema, more commonly involving the parietal and occipital lobes, followed by the frontal lobes, the inferior temporal-occipital junction, and the cerebellum.

- Focal/patchy areas of edema may also be seen in the basal ganglia, brainstem, and deep white matter (external/internal capsules).
- The edema usually reverses completely.
- Hemorrhage (focal hematoma, isolated sulcal/subarachnoid blood or protein) is seen in ~15% of patients.

### ■ Other Imaging Findings

- At catheter angiography and MR angiography, diffuse vasoconstriction, focal vasoconstriction, vasodilatation, and even a string-of-beads appearance have been noted in PRES, consistent with what is typically described as vasospasm or arteritis.

### ✓ Pearls & ✗ Pitfalls

- ✓ Three different hemispheric patterns may be encountered with similar frequency:
  - ✓ Holohemispheric
  - ✓ Superior frontal sulcal
  - ✓ Primary parietal-occipital
- ✓ These likely represent areas of watershed blood supply from the middle, anterior, and posterior cerebral arteries.
- ✗ Focal areas of restricted diffusion (likely representing infarction or tissue injury with cytotoxic edema) are uncommon (11–26%) and may be associated with an adverse outcome.

# Case 96

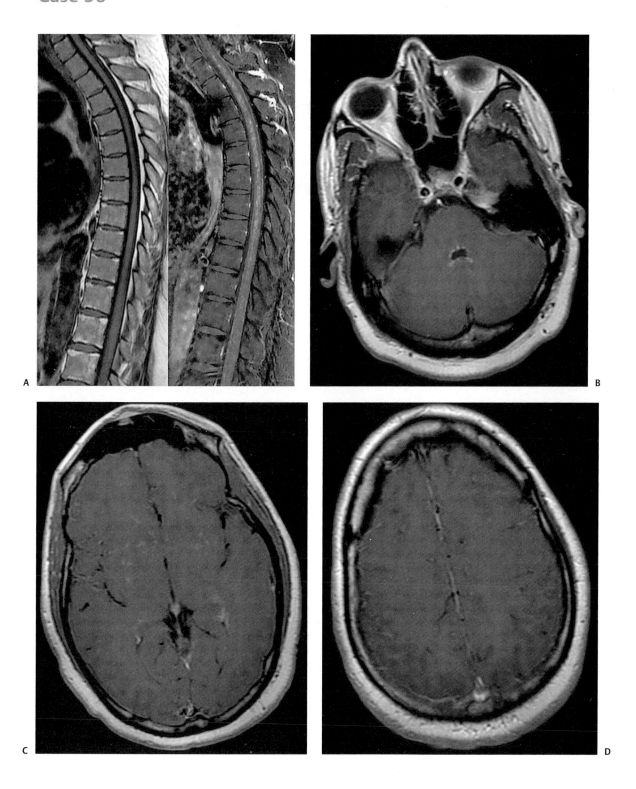

A

B

C

D

## Clinical Presentation

A 43-year-old African-American man with a chronic lung condition presenting with the new onset of seizures.

## ■ Imaging Findings

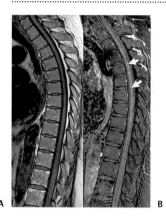
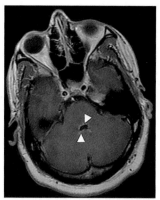
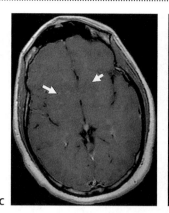
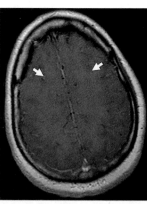

**(A)** Sagittal T1-weighted images (WIs) before and after contrast demonstrate extensive linear leptomeningeal enhancement in the thoracic region (*white arrows*). **(B)** Nodular enhancement around the 4th ventricle is demonstrated in the postcontrast axial T1WI (*arrowheads*). **(C)** Postcontrast axial T1WI shows the distribution of linear and nodular areas of enhancement in the basal ganglia following the Virchow-Robin spaces (*arrows*), which is indicative of leptomeningeal involvement. **(D)** On a postcontrast axial T1WI, leptomeningeal enhancement is also noted in the frontal convexities (*arrows*).

## ■ Differential Diagnosis

- *Leptomeningeal neurosarcoidosis:* Sarcoidosis is a diagnosis of exclusion. It is characterized by nodular or linear enhancement of the cortical sulci, perivascular spaces, and cisterns around the base of the brain.
- *Leptomeningeal carcinomatosis:* Diffuse seeding of the leptomeninges by tumor metastases is known as denominated leptomeningeal carcinomatosis or leptomeningeal disease. It is commonly found in breast carcinoma, lung carcinoma, and melanoma in adults, and in hematogenous malignancies and primitive neuroectodermal tumor in children.
- *Tuberculous meningitis:* In countries with a high incidence of tuberculosis, tuberculous meningitis is typically a disease of young children that develops 3 to 6 months after primary infection. In countries with a low incidence of tuberculosis, tuberculous meningitis commonly affects adults and frequently arises after the reactivation of a dormant subcortical or meningeal focus. Imaging findings include dural thickening, calcifications, meningeal enhancement (predominantly basal), infarcts, and communicating hydrocephalus.

## ■ Essential Facts

- Sarcoidosis is an idiopathic systemic disease histologically characterized by the formation of noncaseating granulomas.
- The clinical presentation includes cranial neuropathy (especially of the optic and facial nerves) and neuroendocrine disorders (e.g., secondary diabetes insipidus); it is symptomatic in fewer than 10% of patients.
- Leptomeningeal enhancement is predominantly basal.
- Small enhancing nodules are seen on the surface of the brain and in the perivascular spaces.
- Diffuse dural thickening or a focal dural mass shows homogeneous contrast enhancement. These lesions are commonly dark on T2WIs.

- Spinal neurosarcoidosis may affect the cord and nerve roots, the intradural-extramedullary space, the intracanalicular-extradural space, and the vertebral bodies and intervertebral disks.
- Leptomeningeal involvement manifests as thin linear leptomeningeal enhancement or small nodules.

## ■ Other Imaging Findings

- Magnetic resonance imaging:
  - Periventricular and deep white matter T2 hyperintensities
  - Multiple or solitary parenchymal masses with a ringlike appearance; enhancement when biologically active
  - Chiasmatic lesions visualized as foci of increased signal intensity on fluid-attenuated inversion recovery images
  - Loss of high T1 signal in the neurohypophysis
- Intramedullary sarcoidosis: nonspecific appearance; fusiform enlargement of the spinal cord in the cervical or upper thoracic levels; high T2 signal, low T1 signal, and patchy enhancement after contrast administration

## ✓ Pearls & ✗ Pitfalls

- ✓ Leptomeningeal sarcoidosis can be distinguished from dural disease by involvement of the cortical sulci, perivascular spaces, cranial nerves, and cisterns around the base of the brain.
- ✓ Sarcoidosis is a diagnosis of exclusion.
- ✗ Enhancing parenchymal lesions contiguous with enhancing meningeal areas may be mistaken for a meningioma.

# Case 97

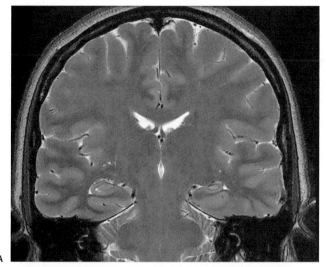

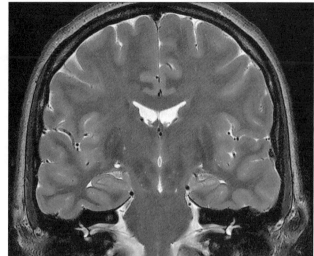

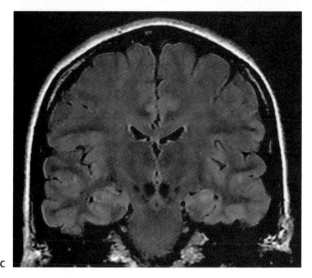

## ▣ Clinical Presentation

A 25-year-old with epilepsy.

## ■ Imaging Findings

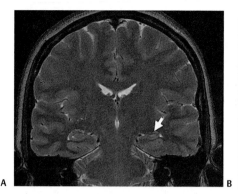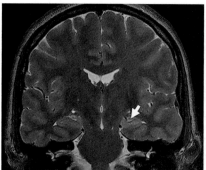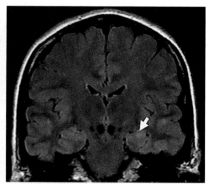

A                            B                            C

**(A,B)** Coronal T2-weighted images (WIs) perpendicular to the long axis of the hippocampus show decreased height of the left hippocampus in comparison with the right and mild architectural distortion (*arrows*). **(C)** Fluid-attenuated inversion recovery coronal image at the level of the hippocampal head shows increased signal on the left in comparison with the right and with the remainder of the temporal cortex (*arrow*).

## ■ Differential Diagnosis

- *Mesial temporal sclerosis (MTS):* Atrophy of one or both hippocampal formations is indicative of MTS. There is increased T2 signal and architectural distortion. The abnormalities may involve other areas of the temporal lobe.
- *Herpes encephalitis:* This is the most common type of sporadic viral encephalitis, with a predilection for the temporal lobes. Magnetic resonance imaging (MRI) shows T2 hyperintensity corresponding to edematous changes in the temporal lobes, inferior frontal lobes, and insula, with a predilection for the medial temporal lobes. Foci of hemorrhage occasionally can be observed on MRI.
- *Cortical dysplasia:* This is defined as a focal abnormal arrangement of neurons and glia in the cortex. Images show distortion in the gray–white matter junction with thickening of the cortex. Mild T2 hyperintensity of the gray matter (cortex) is present. The temporal lobe is most frequently involved, followed by the frontal and occipital lobes.

## ■ Essential Facts

- MTS is the most frequently observed abnormality in temporal lobe epilepsy (TLE).
- Neuronal loss and gliosis, involving principally the hippocampus and/or the amygdala and occasionally extending to other mesial temporal structures (entorhinal cortex and parahippocampal gyrus) or even throughout the temporal lobe, is common.
- Whether MTS is the cause or result of TLE is controversial.
- Patients with TLE often have a history of an initial precipitating injury, usually before the age of 5 years.
- Status epilepticus, especially complicated febrile convulsions, have been associated with hippocampal damage and unilateral sclerosis.

## ■ Other Imaging Findings

- MRI:
  - Thin (1–3 mm) oblique coronal images orthogonal to the long axis of the hippocampus are required.
  - Findings include hippocampal atrophy, increased signal on T2WIs, loss of internal structure, and decreased signal on T1WIs.
  - Additional abnormalities include loss of hippocampal head digitations, enlarged temporal horn, and increased T2 signal in the ipsilateral anterior temporal lobe. The affected hippocampus shows architectural distortion. MTS can also present with atrophy of the ipsilateral amygdala or asymmetry of the fornix.
- Ictal single-photon emission computed tomography (SPECT), with the use of tracers that accumulate and remain "fixed" in different areas of the brain proportional to the regional cerebral blood flow at the time of injection, is an important tool for localizing seizures in a presurgical evaluation.
- Interictal SPECT in focal epilepsy has shown areas of low perfusion in some patients, mainly those with TLE.

## ✓ Pearls & ✘ Pitfalls

- ✓ In 15 to 20% of cases of MTS, another potentially epileptogenic anomaly is found outside the hippocampus (dual pathology).
- ✓ The most common types of lesions outside the hippocampus are developmental abnormalities, such as cortical dysgenesis and gliotic lesions acquired in early childhood.
- ✘ Dilatation of the ipsilateral temporal horn is found to be associated with hippocampal atrophy. Sometimes, temporal horn dilatation is more severe on the side opposite the sclerotic hippocampus. This may be a falsely lateralizing finding.

# Case 98

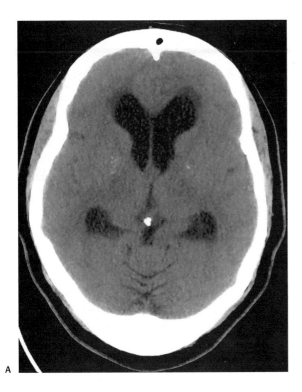

A

## ▣ Clinical Presentation

A 39-year-old woman with intermittent positional headache.

## Further Work-up

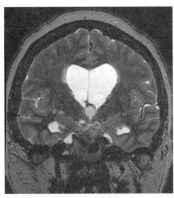

B

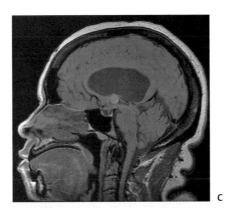

C

D

## ■ Imaging Findings

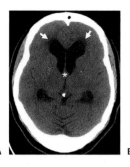
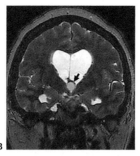
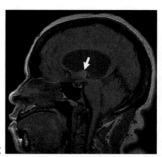
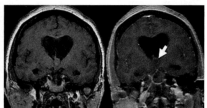

**(A)** Axial computed tomography (CT) demonstrates enlarged frontal horns and transependymal fluid leak (*white arrows*), which is indicative of hydrocephalus. There is a mass with attenuation similar to that of white matter in the vicinity of the foramen of Monro (*asterisk*). **(B)** Coronal T2-weighted image (WI) shows a mass in the superior aspect of the 3rd ventricle (*arrow*), with a central intermediate signal and a thin rim of low signal. **(C)** On the sagittal T1WI, the lesion has increased signal intensity (*arrow*). The lateral ventricles are dilated, whereas the 3rd and 4th are not. **(D)** Coronal T1WIs before and after contrast show no enhancement of the mass (*arrow*).

## ■ Differential Diagnosis

- **Colloid cyst of the 3rd ventricle:** Remnants of Rathke cleft forming a well-defined round mass in the vicinity of the foramen of Monro are indicative of this diagnosis. Obstructive hydrocephalus is common. There is no enhancement after gadolinium injection.
- *Central neurocytoma:* This is a relatively benign tumor arising from neuronal precursor elements. Imaging studies show a well-defined, lobulated intraventricular mass growing near the foramen of Monro or septum pellucidum. There is mild to moderate enhancement. Calcifications and cystic changes are common. Most patients are young adults and can present with symptoms of ventricular obstruction.
- *Intraventricular hemorrhage:* Intraventricular clots may be found in the dependant portion of the ventricle or attached to the ventricular walls. The signal intensity may vary depending on the age of the blood products they contain.

## ■ Essential Facts

- Colloid cysts are rare intracranial lesions.
- Clinical symptoms may be intermittent, self-resolving, and nonspecific.
- Headache is often the presenting symptom. It is described as brief (lasting seconds to minutes) and is initiated, exacerbated, or relieved by a change in position.
- Some colloid cysts result in the acute onset of hydrocephalus and may lead to sudden death.
- A round or oval mass is present in the anterior aspect of the 3rd ventricle.
- Treatment options include simple shunting of both lateral ventricles, open surgical removal, and percutaneous aspiration (simple cyst aspiration, stereotactic aspiration, endoscopic procedure).

## ■ Other Imaging Findings

- On CT scans, the lesions are often hyperdense.
- A thin rim of enhancement after the administration of iodinated contrast material is thought to represent the cyst capsule.
- The magnetic resonance imaging appearance is variable.

## ✓ Pearls & ✗ Pitfalls

- ✓ Because of the attachment of the cyst to the 3rd ventricular roof, the lesion may be pendulous, resulting in intermittent foraminal obstruction.
- ✗ Rarely, colloid cysts may present with rim enhancement.

# Case 99

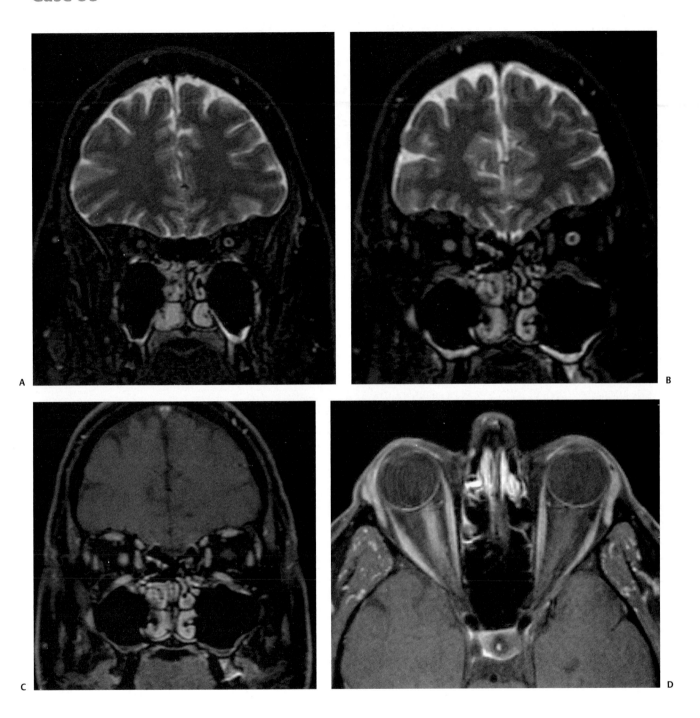

## Clinical Presentation

A 42-year-old woman presenting with unilateral pain, decreased visual acuity, and loss of color vision.

## ■ Imaging Findings

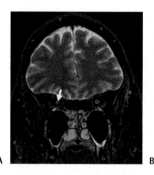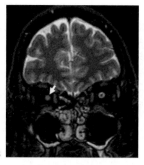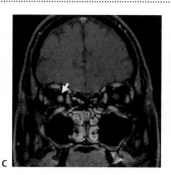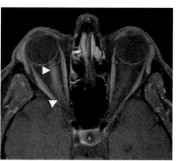

A          B          C          D

**(A,B)** Coronal T2-weighted images (WIs) of the orbits show enlargement of the right optic nerve (*arrow*), resulting in effacement of the right optic nerve sheath in comparison with the left. **(C)** Coronal postcontrast T1WI shows that the right optic nerve is enlarged and enhances homogeneously (*arrow*). **(D)** On the axial T1WI, note how the enhancement extends from the apex of the orbit to the globe (*arrowheads*).

## ■ Differential Diagnosis

- **Optic neuritis:** This is inflammatory optic neuropathy resulting in vision loss. Magnetic resonance imaging (MRI) findings may be normal or demonstrate T2 hyperintensity with a normal or mildly enlarged optic nerve. Contrast enhancement can involve a segment or the entire optic nerve.
- *Sarcoidosis:* This is an inflammatory disorder that may involve any part of the optic pathways, most commonly the optic nerves and optic chiasm. The anterior optic pathways are involved in ~1 to 5% of cases of sarcoidosis. On MRI, there is bilateral optic nerve involvement. Pathologic enhancement of the optic nerve from the globe to the chiasm is strongly suggestive of sarcoidosis. There is enhancement of the frontobasal meninges and enlargement of the lacrimal glands.
- *Idiopathic orbital inflammatory syndrome:* There is localized inflammation within the orbit, resulting in pain, proptosis, and ophthalmoparesis. On MRI, there is enlargement of multiple muscles, irregular borders with extension to the orbital fat, and enhancement around the globe. There are mass lesions that are hypointense to orbital fat on T1WIs and isointense or minimally hyperintense to fat on T2WIs.

## ■ Essential Facts

- Optic neuritis is one of the most common causes of acute visual loss in young adults.
- Most cases are the result of idiopathic inflammatory demyelination.
- The risk for the development of multiple sclerosis after an episode of optic neuritis is ~40% after 10 years and 50% after 20 years.
- Acute optic neuritis associated with transverse myelitis is known as neuromyelitis optica or Devic syndrome.

- Optic neuritis also may occur in isolation or secondary to sarcoidosis, viral infection (including human immunodeficiency virus–related optic neuropathy), vasculitides, ischemia, toxins, or radiation.
- Clinically silent white matter lesions within the brain are often seen at the time of the presentation of optic neuritis.

## ■ Other Imaging Findings

- MRI:
  - T2 hyperintensity and contrast enhancement involving segments of the entire length of the optic nerve and extending posteriorly to involve the optic chiasm
  - Enhancement of the nerve sheath
  - Distension of the nerve sheath anteriorly
  - Continued atrophy of the optic nerve over months and years after the episode of optic neuritis

## ✓ Pearls & ✗ Pitfalls

- ✓ The real contribution of imaging in the setting of optic neuritis is the imaging of the brain, not the optic nerves themselves.
- ✗ False-positive results in orbital imaging can result from failure of complete fat saturation related to magnetic susceptibility artifact resulting from dental amalgam and air–soft tissue interfaces, particularly at the inferior margin of the orbit.

# Case 100

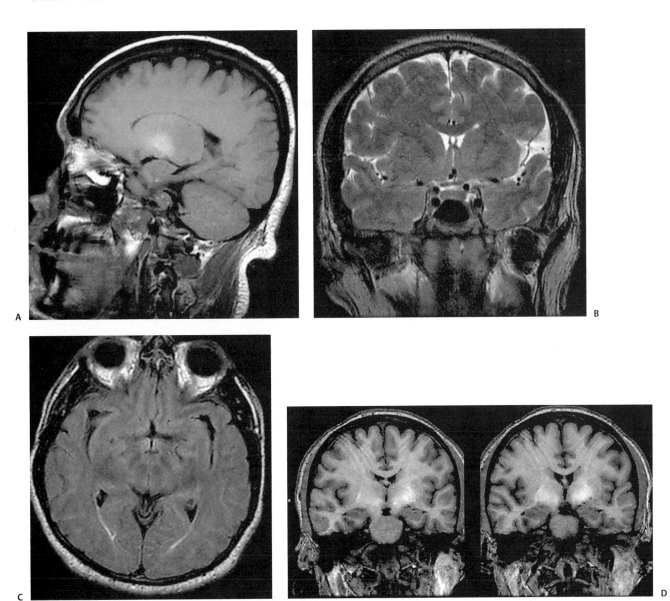

## Clinical Presentation

A 37-year-old man with cirrhosis presents with rigidity and an acute confusional state.

### ■ Imaging Findings

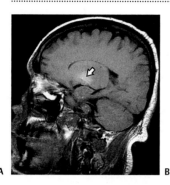
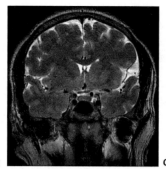
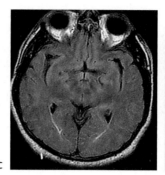
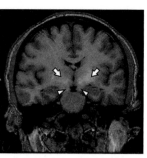

**(A)** Sagittal T1-weighted image (WI) shows increased T1 signal in the globus pallidus (*arrow*). **(B)** Coronal T2WI shows normal signal in the globus pallidus. **(C)** Axial fluid-attenuated inversion recovery (FLAIR) image shows no abnormal signal. **(D)** Coronal T1WI shows increased signal bilaterally in the globus pallidus (*arrows*) and in the substantia nigra (*arrowheads*).

### ■ Differential Diagnosis

- **Hepatic encephalopathy:** Liver dysfunction causes a spectrum of neuropsychiatric abnormalities. Imaging studies show increased signal on T1WIs in the globus pallidus bilaterally, diffuse brain edema, and diffuse increased signal of the hemispheric white matter on FLAIR images. No contrast enhancement is present.
- **Total parenteral nutrition (TPN):** Manganese deposits in the globus pallidus are seen in patients on TPN. The findings are similar to those in hepatic encephalopathy.
- **Nonketotic hyperglycemic episode:** The imaging findings are the same as those in hepatic encephalopathy.

### ■ Essential Facts

- The T1 hyperintensities are caused by manganese deposits, which have neurotoxic effects.
- Manganese is more prominent in the medial segment of the globus pallidus, followed by the substantia nigra pars reticulata.
- White matter abnormalities are present, related to an increased concentration of ammonia in the central nervous system.
- These findings can be reversed after the normalization of liver function.

### ■ Other Imaging Findings

- Computed tomography does not show the abnormalities in the basal ganglia.
- FLAIR images show diffuse hyperintensities in the periventricular hemispheric white matter.
- Magnetic resonance spectroscopy can detect increased glutamine signal and decreased myoinositol.

### ✓ Pearls & ✗ Pitfalls

- ✓ The globus pallidus and white matter lesions can decrease 1 year after liver transplant.
- ✗ Acute hepatic encephalopathy can present with diffuse brain edema and blurring of the gray–white matter junction.

# Further Readings

## Case 1

Alden TD, Ojemann JG, Park TS. Surgical treatment of Chiari I malformation: indications and approaches [review]. Neurosurg Focus 2001;11(1):E2

Schijman E. History, anatomic forms, and pathogenesis of Chiari I malformations. Childs Nerv Syst 2004;20(5):323–328

## Case 2

Rollins N, Joglar J, Perlman J, Chiari II. Coexistent holoprosencephaly and Chiari II malformation. AJNR Am J Neuroradiol 1999;20(9):1678–1681

Wolpert SM, Anderson M, Scott RM, Kwan ES, Runge VM. Chiari II malformation: MR imaging evaluation. AJR Am J Roentgenol 1987;149(5):1033–1042

## Case 3

Patel S, Barkovich AJ. Analysis and classification of cerebellar malformations. AJNR Am J Neuroradiol 2002;23(7):1074–1087

## Case 4

Barkovich AJ, Norman D. Anomalies of the corpus callosum: correlation with further anomalies of the brain. AJR Am J Roentgenol 1988;151(1):171–179

Hetts SW, Sherr EH, Chao S, Gobuty S, Barkovich AJ. Anomalies of the corpus callosum: an MR analysis of the phenotypic spectrum of associated malformations. AJR Am J Roentgenol 2006;187(5):1343–1348

## Case 5

Cecil KM. MR spectroscopy of metabolic disorders. Neuroimaging Clin N Am 2006;16(1):87–116, viii

Cheon JE, Kim IO, Hwang YS, et al. Leukodystrophy in children: a pictorial review of MR imaging features. Radiographics 2002;22(3):461–476

## Case 6

Kiymaz N, Cirak B. Central nervous system lipomas. Tohoku J Exp Med 2002;198(3):203–206

Truwit CL, Barkovich AJ. Pathogenesis of intracranial lipoma: an MR study in 42 patients. AJR Am J Roentgenol 1990;155(4):855–864, discussion 865

## Case 7

Kannegieter LS, Dietrich RB, Pais MJ, Goldenberg TM. Pediatric case of the day. Chiari III malformation. Radiographics 1994;14(2):452–454

Otsubo Y, Sato H, Sato N, Ito H. Cephaloceles and abnormal venous drainage. Childs Nerv Syst 1999;15(6-7):329–332

## Case 8

Ghai S, Fong KW, Toi A, Chitayat D, Pantazi S, Blaser S. Prenatal US and MR imaging findings of lissencephaly: review of fetal cerebral sulcal development. Radiographics 2006;26(2):389–405

Rollins N, Reyes T, Chia J. Diffusion tensor imaging in lissencephaly. AJNR Am J Neuroradiol 2005;26(6):1583–1586

## Case 9

Barkovich AJ, Raybaud CA. Neuroimaging in disorders of cortical development. Neuroimaging Clin N Am 2004;14(2):231–254, viii

## Case 10

Denis D, Chateil JF, Brun M, et al. Schizencephaly: clinical and imaging features in 30 infantile cases. Brain Dev 2000;22(8):475–483

Hayashi N, Tsutsumi Y, Barkovich AJ. Morphological features and associated anomalies of schizencephaly in the clinical population: detailed analysis of MR images. Neuroradiology 2002;44(5):418–427

## Case 11

Albayram S, Melhem ER, Mori S, Zinreich SJ, Barkovich AJ, Kinsman SL. Holoprosencephaly in children: diffusion tensor MR imaging of white matter tracts of the brainstem—initial experience. Radiology 2002;223(3):645–651

Castillo M, Bouldin TW, Scatliff JH, Suzuki K. Radiologic-pathologic correlation. Alobar holoprosencephaly. AJNR Am J Neuroradiol 1993;14(5):1151–1156

Demyer W, Zeman W, Palmer CG. The face predicts the brain: diagnostic significance of median facial anomalies for holoprosencephaly (arhinencephaly). Pediatrics 1964;34:256–263

Simon EM, Hevner R, Pinter JD, et al. Assessment of the deep gray nuclei in holoprosencephaly. AJNR Am J Neuroradiol 2000;21(10):1955–1961

## Case 12

Barkovich AJ, Fram EK, Norman D. Septo-optic dysplasia: MR imaging. Radiology 1989;171(1):189–192

Barkovich AJ, Norman D. Absence of the septum pellucidum: a useful sign in the diagnosis of congenital brain malformations. AJR Am J Roentgenol 1989;152(2):353–360

Smith MM, Strottmann JM. Imaging of the optic nerve and visual pathways. Semin Ultrasound CT MR 2001;22(6):473–487

## Case 13

DiMario FJ Jr, Ramsby G. Magnetic resonance imaging lesion analysis in neurofibromatosis type 1. Arch Neurol 1998;55(4):500–505

Gonen O, Wang ZJ, Viswanathan AK, Molloy PT, Zimmerman RA. Three-dimensional multivoxel proton MR spectroscopy of the brain in children with neurofibromatosis type 1. AJNR Am J Neuroradiol 1999;20(7):1333–1341

Restrepo CS, Riascos RF, Hatta AA, Rojas R. Neurofibromatosis type 1: spinal manifestations of a systemic disease. J Comput Assist Tomogr 2005;29(4):532–539

Shu HH, Mirowitz SA, Wippold FJ II. Neurofibromatosis: MR imaging findings involving the head and spine. AJR Am J Roentgenol 1993;160(1):159–164

## Case 14

Farrell CJ, Plotkin SR. Genetic causes of brain tumors: neurofibromatosis, tuberous sclerosis, von Hippel-Lindau, and other syndromes. Neurol Clin 2007;25(4):925–946, viii

## Case 15

Baron Y, Barkovich AJ. MR imaging of tuberous sclerosis in neonates and young infants. AJNR Am J Neuroradiol 1999;20(5):907–916

Kalantari BN, Salamon N. Neuroimaging of tuberous sclerosis: spectrum of pathologic findings and frontiers in imaging. AJR Am J Roentgenol 2008;190(5):W304–9

Wong V, Khong P-L. Tuberous sclerosis complex: correlation of magnetic resonance imaging (MRI) findings with comorbidities. J Child Neurol 2006;21(2):99–105

## Case 16

Griffiths PD. Sturge-Weber syndrome revisited: the role of neuroradiology. Neuropediatrics 1996;27(6):284–294

Smirniotopoulos JG. Neuroimaging of phakomatoses: Sturge-Weber syndrome, tuberous sclerosis, von Hippel-Lindau syndrome. Neuroimaging Clin N Am 2004;14(2):171–183, vii

## Case 17

Farrell CJ, Plotkin SR. Genetic causes of brain tumors: neurofibromatosis, tuberous sclerosis, von Hippel-Lindau, and other syndromes. Neurol Clin 2007;25(4):925–946, viii

Leung RS, Biswas SV, Duncan M, Rankin S. Imaging features of von Hippel-Lindau disease. Radiographics 2008;28(1):65–79, quiz 323

## Case 18

Evans A, Stoodley N, Halpin S. Magnetic resonance imaging of intraspinal cystic lesions: a pictorial review. Curr Probl Diagn Radiol 2002;31(3):79–94

Greitz D. Unraveling the riddle of syringomyelia. Neurosurg Rev 2006;29(4):251–263, discussion 264

## Case 19

Han JS, Benson JE, Kaufman B, et al. Demonstration of diastematomyelia and associated abnormalities with MR imaging. AJNR Am J Neuroradiol 1985;6(2):215–219

Kaffenberger DA, Heinz ER, Oakes JW, Boyko O. Meningocele manqué: radiologic findings with clinical correlation. AJNR Am J Neuroradiol 1992;13(4):1083–1088

Tortori-Donati P, Rossi A, Biancheri R, Cama A. Magnetic resonance imaging of spinal dysraphism. Top Magn Reson Imaging 2001;12(6):375–409

## Case 20

Diel J, Ortiz O, Losada RA, Price DB, Hayt MW, Katz DS. The sacrum: pathologic spectrum, multimodality imaging, and subspecialty approach. Radiographics 2001;21(1):83–104

Tortori-Donati P, Rossi A, Biancheri R, Cama A. Magnetic resonance imaging of spinal dysraphism. Top Magn Reson Imaging 2001;12(6):375–409

## Case 21

Koeller KK, Rushing EJ. From the archives of the AFIP: Oligodendroglioma and its variants: radiologic-pathologic correlation. Radiographics 2005;25(6):1669–1688

White ML, Zhang Y, Kirby P, Ryken TC. Can tumor contrast enhancement be used as a criterion for differentiating tumor grades of oligodendrogliomas? AJNR Am J Neuroradiol 2005;26(4):784–790

## Case 22

Daumas-Duport C, Scheithauer BW, Chodkiewicz JP, Laws ER Jr, Vedrenne C. Dysembryoplastic neuroepithelial tumor: a surgically curable tumor of young patients with intractable partial seizures. Report of thirty-nine cases. Neurosurgery 1988;23(5):545–556

Fernandez C, Girard N, Paz Paredes A, Bouvier-Labit C, Lena G, Figarella-Branger D. The usefulness of MR imaging in the diagnosis of dysembryoplastic neuroepithelial tumor in children: a study of 14 cases. AJNR Am J Neuroradiol 2003;24(5):829–834

Shin JH, Lee HK, Khang SK, et al. Neuronal tumors of the central nervous system: radiologic findings and pathologic correlation. Radiographics 2002;22(5):1177–1189

## Case 23

Brown JY, Morokoff AP, Mitchell PJ, Gonzales MF. Unusual imaging appearance of an intracranial dermoid cyst. AJNR Am J Neuroradiol 2001;22(10):1970–1972

Osborn AG, Preece MT. Intracranial cysts: radiologic-pathologic correlation and imaging approach. Radiology 2006;239(3):650–664

## Case 24

Chen C-Y, Wong J-S, Hsieh S-C, Chu J-S, Chan WP. Intracranial epidermoid cyst with hemorrhage: MR imaging findings. AJNR Am J Neuroradiol 2006;27(2):427–429

Ochi M, Hayashi K, Hayashi T, et al. Unusual CT and MR appearance of an epidermoid tumor of the cerebellopontine angle. AJNR Am J Neuroradiol 1998;19(6):1113–1115

Tsuruda JS, Chew WM, Moseley ME, Norman D. Diffusion-weighted MR imaging of the brain: value of differentiating between extraaxial cysts and epidermoid tumors. AJNR Am J Neuroradiol 1990;11(5):925–931, discussion 932–934

## Case 25

Bonneville F, Sarrazin J-L, Marsot-Dupuch K, et al. Unusual lesions of the cerebellopontine angle: a segmental approach. Radiographics 2001;21(2):419–438

Koeller KK, Sandberg GD; Armed Forces Institute of Pathology. From the archives of the AFIP. Cerebral intraventricular neoplasms: radiologic-pathologic correlation. Radiographics 2002;22(6):1473–1505

## Case 26

Koeller KK, Rushing EJ. From the archives of the AFIP: medulloblastoma: a comprehensive review with radiologic-pathologic correlation. Radiographics 2003;23(6):1613–1637

Stavrou T, Dubovsky EC, Reaman GH, Goldstein AM, Vezina G. Intracranial calcifications in childhood medulloblastoma: relation to nevoid basal cell carcinoma syndrome. AJNR Am J Neuroradiol 2000;21(4):790–794

## Case 27

Coates TL, Hinshaw DB Jr, Peckman N, et al. Pediatric choroid plexus neoplasms: MR, CT, and pathologic correlation. Radiology 1989;173(1):81–88

Koeller KK, Sandberg GD; Armed Forces Institute of Pathology. From the archives of the AFIP. Cerebral intraventricular neoplasms: radiologic-pathologic correlation. Radiographics 2002;22(6):1473–1505

## Case 28

Ho VB, Smirniotopoulos JG, Murphy FM, Rushing EJ. Radiologic-pathologic correlation: hemangioblastoma. AJNR Am J Neuroradiol 1992;13(5):1343–1352

Lee SR, Sanches J, Mark AS, Dillon WP, Norman D, Newton TH. Posterior fossa hemangioblastomas: MR imaging. Radiology 1989;171(2):463–468

Slater A, Moore NR, Huson SM. The natural history of cerebellar hemangioblastomas in von Hippel-Lindau disease. AJNR Am J Neuroradiol 2003;24(8):1570–1574

Vilanova JC, Barceló J, Smirniotopoulos JG, et al. Hemangioma from head to toe: MR imaging with pathologic correlation. Radiographics 2004;24(2):367–385

## Case 29

Barkovich AJ, Newton TH. MR of aqueductal stenosis: evidence of a broad spectrum of tectal distortion. AJNR Am J Neuroradiol 1989;10(3):471–476

Friedman DP. Extrapineal abnormalities of the tectal region: MR imaging findings. AJR Am J Roentgenol 1992;159(4):859–866

## Case 30

Koeller KK, Rushing EJ. From the archives of the AFIP: pilocytic astrocytoma: radiologic-pathologic correlation. Radiographics 2004;24(6):1693–1708

Lee YY, Van Tassel P, Bruner JM, Moser RP, Share JC. Juvenile pilocytic astrocytomas: CT and MR characteristics. AJR Am J Roentgenol 1989;152(6):1263–1270

## Case 31

Meijer OWM, Weijmans EJ, Knol DL, et al. Tumor-volume changes after radiosurgery for vestibular schwannoma: implications for follow-up MR imaging protocol. AJNR Am J Neuroradiol 2008;29(5):906–910

## Case 32

Pope WB, Sayre J, Perlina A, Villablanca JP, Mischel PS, Cloughesy TF. MR imaging correlates of survival in patients with high-grade gliomas. AJNR Am J Neuroradiol 2005;26(10):2466–2474

Rees JH, Smirniotopoulos JG, Jones RV, Wong K. Glioblastoma multiforme: radiologic-pathologic correlation. Radiographics 1996;16(6):1413–1438, quiz 1462–1463

## Case 33

Banks KP, Brown SJ. AJR teaching file: solid masses of the pineal region. AJR Am J Roentgenol 2006;186(3 Suppl):S233–S235

Smirniotopoulos JG, Rushing EJ, Mena H. Pineal region masses: differential diagnosis. Radiographics 1992;12(3):577–596

## Case 34

Buetow MP, Buetow PC, Smirniotopoulos JG. Typical, atypical, and misleading features in meningioma. Radiographics 1991;11(6):1087–1106

Nagar VA, Ye JR, Ng WH, et al. Diffusion-weighted MR imaging: diagnosing atypical or malignant meningiomas and detecting tumor dedifferentiation. AJNR Am J Neuroradiol 2008;29(6):1147–1152

Toh C-H, Castillo M, Wong AM-C, et al. Differentiation between classic and atypical meningiomas with use of diffusion tensor imaging. AJNR Am J Neuroradiol 2008;29(9):1630–1635

## Case 35

Chacko AG, Chacko G, Seshadri MS, Chandy MJ. The 'capsule' of pituitary macroadenomas represents normal pituitary gland: a histopathological study. Br J Neurosurg 2003;17(3):213–218

Tokumaru AM, Sakata I, Terada H, Kosuda S, Nawashiro H, Yoshii M. Optic nerve hyperintensity on T2-weighted images among patients with pituitary macroadenoma: correlation with visual impairment. AJNR Am J Neuroradiol 2006;27(2):250–254

Tosaka M, Sato N, Hirato J, et al. Assessment of hemorrhage in pituitary macroadenoma by T2*-weighted gradient-echo MR imaging. AJNR Am J Neuroradiol 2007;28(10):2023–2029

## Case 36

Koeller KK, Rosenblum RS, Morrison AL. Neoplasms of the spinal cord and filum terminale: radiologic-pathologic correlation. Radiographics 2000;20(6):1721–1749

## Case 37

Krol G, Sze G, Malkin M, Walker R. MR of cranial and spinal meningeal carcinomatosis: comparison with CT and myelography. AJR Am J Roentgenol 1988;151(3):583–588

## Case 38

Armao D, Castillo M, Chen H, Kwock L. Colloid cyst of the third ventricle: imaging-pathologic correlation. AJNR Am J Neuroradiol 2000;21(8):1470–1477

Maeder PP, Holtås SL, Basibüyük LN, Salford LG, Tapper UA, Brun A. Colloid cysts of the third ventricle: correlation of MR and CT findings with histology and chemical analysis. AJR Am J Roentgenol 1990;155(1):135–141

## Case 39

Breger RK, Williams AL, Daniels DL, et al. Contrast enhancement in spinal MR imaging. AJR Am J Roentgenol 1989;153(2):387–391

Shrier DA, Rubio A, Numaguchi Y, Powers JM. Infarcted spinal schwannoma: an unusual MR finding. AJNR Am J Neuroradiol 1996;17(8):1566–1568

## Case 40

Choi SH, Kwon BJ, Na DG, Kim JH, Han MH, Chang KH. Pituitary adenoma, craniopharyngioma, and Rathke cleft cyst involving both intrasellar and suprasellar regions: differentiation using MRI. Clin Radiol 2007;62(5):453–462

Garnett MR, Puget S, Grill J, Sainte-Rose C. Craniopharyngioma. Orphanet J Rare Dis 2007;2:18

## Case 41

Hammoud DA, Wasserman BA. Diffuse axonal injuries: pathophysiology and imaging. Neuroimaging Clin N Am 2002;12(2):205–216

Zheng WB, Liu GR, Li LP, Wu RH. Prediction of recovery from a post-traumatic coma state by diffusion-weighted imaging (DWI) in patients with diffuse axonal injury. Neuroradiology 2007;49(3):271–279

## Case 42

Parizel PM, Van Goethem JW, Özsarlak Ö, Maes M, Phillips CD. New developments in the neuroradiological diagnosis of craniocerebral trauma. Eur Radiol 2005;15(3):569–581

## Case 43

Provenzale JCT. CT and MR imaging of acute cranial trauma. Emerg Radiol 2007;14(1):1–12

## Case 44

Toyama Y, Kobayashi T, Nishiyama Y, Satoh K, Ohkawa M, Seki K. CT for acute stage of closed head injury. Radiat Med 2005;23(5):309–316

## Case 45

Hardman JM, Manoukian A. Pathology of head trauma. Neuroimaging Clin N Am 2002;12(2):175–187, vii

## Case 46

Young RJ, Destian S. Imaging of traumatic intracranial hemorrhage. Neuroimaging Clin N Am 2002;12(2):189–204

## Case 47

Van Goethem JW, Maes M, Özsarlak O, van den HauweL, ParizelPM. Imaging in spinal trauma. Eur Radiol 2005;15(3):582–590

## Case 48

Chang FC, Lirng JF, Luo CB, et al. Evaluation of clinical and MR findings for the prognosis of spinal epidural haematomas. Clin Radiol 2005;60(7):762–770

Kebaish KM, Awad JN. Spinal epidural hematoma causing acute cauda equina syndrome. Neurosurg Focus 2004;16(6):e1

## Case 49

Demaerel P. Magnetic resonance imaging of spinal cord trauma: a pictorial essay. Neuroradiology 2006;48(4):223–232

Van Goethem JW, Maes M, Özsarlak O, van den Hauwe L, Parizel PM. Imaging in spinal trauma. Eur Radiol 2005;15(3):582–590

## Case 50

Barnes PD, Krasnokutsky M. Imaging of the central nervous system in suspected or alleged nonaccidental injury, including the mimics. Top Magn Reson Imaging 2007;18(1):53–74

Lonergan GJ, Baker AM, Morey MK, Boos SC. From the archives of the AFIP. Child abuse: radiologic-pathologic correlation. Radiographics 2003;23(4):811–845

## Case 51

Connor SE, Chaudhary N. Imaging of maxillofacial and skull base trauma. Imaging 2007;19:71–82

Kerman M, Cirak B, Dagtekin A. Management of skull base fractures. Neurosurg Q 2002;12:23–41

Larsen DW. Traumatic vascular injuries and their management. Neuroimaging Clin N Am 2002;12(2):249–269

## Case 52

Johnson PL, Eckard DA, Chason DP, Brecheisen MA, Batnitzky S. Imaging of acquired cerebral herniations. Neuroimaging Clin N Am 2002;12(2):217–228

## Case 53

Sundgren PC, Philipp M, Maly PV. Spinal trauma. Neuroimaging Clin N Am 2007;17(1):73–85

## Case 54

Leone A, Guglielmi G, Cassar-Pullicino VN, Bonomo L. Lumbar intervertebral instability: a review. Radiology 2007;245(1):62–77

Ulmer JL, Mathews VP, Elster AD, King JC. Lumbar spondylolysis without spondylolisthesis: recognition of isolated posterior element subluxation on sagittal MR. AJNR Am J Neuroradiol 1995;16(7):1393–1398

## Case 55

Green JD, Harle TS, Harris JH Jr. Anterior subluxation of the cervical spine: hyperflexion sprain. AJNR Am J Neuroradiol 1981;2(3):243–250

Lingawi SS. The naked facet sign. Radiology 2001;219(2):366–367

Shanmuganathan K, Mirvis SE, Levine AM. Rotational injury of cervical facets: CT analysis of fracture patterns with implications for management and neurologic outcome. AJR Am J Roentgenol 1994;163(5):1165–1169

Yetkin Z, Osborn AG, Giles DS, Haughton VM. Uncovertebral and facet joint dislocations in cervical articular pillar fractures: CT evaluation. AJNR Am J Neuroradiol 1985;6(4):633–637

## Case 56

Flis CM, Jäger HR, Sidhu PS. Carotid and vertebral artery dissections: clinical aspects, imaging features and endovascular treatment. Eur Radiol 2007;17(3):820–834

Shin JH, Suh DC, Choi CG, Leei HK. Vertebral artery dissection: spectrum of imaging findings with emphasis on angiography and correlation with clinical presentation. Radiographics 2000;20(6):1687–1696

## Case 57

Brisman JL, Song JK, Newell DW. Cerebral aneurysms. N Engl J Med 2006;355(9):928–939

Gilbert ME, Sergott RC. Intracranial aneurysms. Curr Opin Ophthalmol 2006;17(6):513–518

van Gijn J, Kerr RS, Rinkel GJ. Subarachnoid haemorrhage. Lancet 2007;369(9558):306–318

## Case 58

Chiu D, Shedden P, Bratina P, Grotta JC. Clinical features of moyamoya disease in the United States. Stroke 1998;29(7):1347–1351

Togao O, Mihara F, Yoshiura T, et al. Cerebral hemodynamics in Moyamoya disease: correlation between perfusion-weighted MR imaging and cerebral angiography. AJNR Am J Neuroradiol 2006;27(2):391–397

## Case 59

Elbers J, Benseler SM. Central nervous system vasculitis in children. Curr Opin Rheumatol 2008;20(1):47–54

Küker W. Cerebral vasculitis: imaging signs revisited. Neuroradiology 2007;49(6):471–479

## Case 60

De Monyé C, Dippel DW, Dijkshoorn ML, et al. MDCT Detection of Fibromuscular Dysplasia of the Internal Carotid Artery. AJR Am J Roentgenol 2007;188(4):W367-W369

Plouin PF, Perdu J, La Batide-Alanore A, Boutouyrie P, Gimenez-Roqueplo AP, Jeunemaitre X. Fibromuscular dysplasia. Orphanet J Rare Dis 2007;2:28

## Case 61

Cormier PJ, Long ER, Russell EJ. MR imaging of posterior fossa infarctions: vascular territories and clinical correlates. Radiographics 1992;12(6):1079–1096

Piechowski-Jówiak B, Boggouslavsky J. Vascular disorders of the posterior circulation – an anatomico-clinical overview. Adv Clin Neurosci Rehabil 2004;4:6–9

## Case 62

Yamada M, Yoshimura S, Kaku Y, et al. Prediction of neurologic deterioration in patients with lacunar infarction in the territory of the lenticulostriate artery using perfusion CT. AJNR Am J Neuroradiol 2004;25(3):402–408

## Case 63

Blitstein MK, Tung GA. MRI of cerebral microhemorrhages. AJR Am J Roentgenol 2007;189(3):720–725

Chao CP, Kotsenas AL, Broderick DF. Cerebral amyloid angiopathy: CT and MR imaging findings. Radiographics 2006;26(5):1517–1531

## Case 64

Leach JL, Fortuna RB, Jones BV, Gaskill-Shipley MF. Imaging of cerebral venous thrombosis: current techniques, spectrum of findings, and diagnostic pitfalls. Radiographics 2006;26(suppl 1):S19–S41, discussion S42–S43

Lee SK, terBrugge KG. Cerebral venous thrombosis in adults: the role of imaging evaluation and management. Neuroimaging Clin N Am 2003;13(1):139–152

## Case 65

Camacho DL, Smith JK, Grimme JD, Keyserling HF, Castillo M. Atypical MR imaging perfusion in developmental venous anomalies. AJNR Am J Neuroradiol 2004;25(9):1549–1552

Rivera PP, Willinsky RA, Porter PJ. Intracranial cavernous malformations. Neuroimaging Clin N Am 2003;13(1):27–40

## Case 66

Hartmann A, Mast H, Mohr JP, et al. Determinants of staged endovascular and surgical treatment outcome of brain arteriovenous malformations. Stroke 2005;36(11):2431–2435

Stapf C, Khaw AV, Sciacca RR, et al. Effect of age on clinical and morphological characteristics in patients with brain arteriovenous malformation. Stroke 2003;34(11):2664–2669

## Case 67

Berenstein A, Lasjaunias P. Surgical Neuroangiography. New York: Springer;1993

Jones BV, Ball WS, Tomsick TA, Millard J, Crone KR. Vein of Galen aneurysmal malformation: diagnosis and treatment of 13 children with extended clinical follow-up. AJNR Am J Neuroradiol 2002;23(10):1717–1724

Mitchell PJ, Rosenfeld JV, Dargaville P, et al. Endovascular management of vein of Galen aneurysmal malformations presenting in the neonatal period. AJNR Am J Neuroradiol 2001;22(7):1403–1409

## Case 68

Derdeyn CP. Mechanisms of ischemic stroke secondary to large artery atherosclerotic disease. Neuroimaging Clin N Am 2007;17(3):303–311, vii–viii

Romero JM, Ackerman RH, Dault NA, Lev MH. Noninvasive evaluation of carotid artery stenosis: indications, strategies, and accuracy. Neuroimaging Clin N Am 2005;15(2):351–365, xi

## Case 69

Andersson T, van Dijk JM, Willinsky RA. Venous manifestations of spinal arteriovenous fistulas. Neuroimaging Clin N Am 2003;13(1):73–93

Krings T, Lasjaunias PL, Hans FJ, et al. Imaging in spinal vascular disease. Neuroimaging Clin N Am 2007;17(1):57–72

## Case 70

Kremer S, Abu Eid M, Bierry G, et al. Accuracy of delayed post-contrast FLAIR MR imaging for the diagnosis of leptomeningeal infectious or tumoral diseases. J Neuroradiol 2006;33(5):285–291

Smirniotopoulos JG, Murphy FM, Rushing EJ, Rees JH, Schroeder JW. Patterns of contrast enhancement in the brain and meninges. Radiographics 2007;27(2):525–551

## Case 71

Hermann K-GA, Althoff CE, Schneider U, et al. Spinal changes in patients with spondyloarthritis: comparison of MR imaging and radiographic appearances. Radiographics 2005;25(3):559–569, discussion 569–570

Ledermann HP, Schweitzer ME, Morrison WB, Carrino JA. MR imaging findings in spinal infections: rules or myths? Radiology 2003;228(2):506–514

Stumpe KDM, Zanetti M, Weishaupt D, Hodler J, Boos N, Von Schulthess GK. FDG positron emission tomography for differentiation of degenerative and infectious endplate abnormalities in the lumbar spine detected on MR imaging. AJR Am J Roentgenol 2002;179(5):1151–1157

## Case 72

Leonard JR, Moran CJ, Cross DT III, Wippold FJ II, Schlesinger Y, Storch GA. MR imaging of herpes simplex type 1 encephalitis in infants and young children: a separate pattern of findings. AJR Am J Roentgenol 2000;174(6):1651–1655

Sämann PG, Schlegel J, Müller G, Prantl F, Emminger C, Auer DP. Serial proton MR spectroscopy and diffusion imaging findings in HIV-related herpes simplex encephalitis. AJNR Am J Neuroradiol 2003;24(10):2015–2019

Ukisu R, Kushihashi T, Tanaka E, et al. Diffusion-weighted MR imaging of early-stage Creutzfeldt-Jakob disease: typical and atypical manifestations. Radiographics 2006;26(suppl 1):S191–S204

## Case 73

Kamra P, Azad R, Prasad KN, Jha S, Pradhan S, Gupta RK. Infectious meningitis: prospective evaluation with magnetization transfer MRI. Br J Radiol 2004;77(917):387–394

## Case 74

Camacho DLA, Smith JK, Castillo M. Differentiation of toxoplasmosis and lymphoma in AIDS patients by using apparent diffusion coefficients. AJNR Am J Neuroradiol 2003;24(4):633–637

Smith AB, Smirniotopoulos JG, Rushing EJ. From the archives of the AFIP: central nervous system infections associated with human immunodeficiency virus infection: radiologic-pathologic correlation. Radiographics 2008;28(7):2033–2058

## Case 75

Smith AB, Smirniotopoulos JG, Rushing EJ. From the archives of the AFIP: central nervous system infections associated with human immunodeficiency virus infection: radiologic-pathologic correlation. Radiographics 2008;28(7):2033–2058

Thurnher MM, Post MJ, Rieger A, Kleibl-Popov C, Loewe C, Schindler E. Initial and follow-up MR imaging findings in AIDS-related progressive multifocal leukoencephalopathy treated with highly active antiretroviral therapy. AJNR Am J Neuroradiol 2001;22(5):977–984

## Case 76

Sibtain NA, Chinn RJS. Imaging of the central nervous system in HIV infection. Imaging 2002;14(1):48–59

Smith AB, Smirniotopoulos JG, Rushing EJ. From the archives of the AFIP: central nervous system infections associated with human immunodeficiency virus infection: radiologic-pathologic correlation. Radiographics 2008;28(7):2033–2058

Whiteman ML, Post MJ, Berger JR, Tate LG, Bell MD, Limonte LP. Progressive multifocal leukoencephalopathy in 47 HIV-seropositive patients: neuroimaging with clinical and pathologic correlation. Radiology 1993;187(1):233–240

## Case 77

Smirniotopoulos JG, Murphy FM, Rushing EJ, Rees JH, Schroeder JW. Patterns of contrast enhancement in the brain and meninges. Radiographics 2007;27(2):525–551

## Case 78

Eastwood JD, Vollmer RT, Provenzale JM. Diffusion-weighted imaging in a patient with vertebral and epidural abscesses. AJNR Am J Neuroradiol 2002;23(3):496–498

Numaguchi Y, Rigamonti D, Rothman MI, Sato S, Mihara F, Sadato N. Spinal epidural abscess: evaluation with gadolinium-enhanced MR imaging. Radiographics 1993;13(3):545–559, discussion 559–560

## Case 79

Harisinghani MG, McLoud TC, Shepard J-AO, Ko JP, Shroff MM, Mueller PR. Tuberculosis from head to toe. Radiographics 2000;20(2):449–470, quiz 528–529, 532

Jung NY, Jee WH, Ha KY, Park CK, Byun JY. Discrimination of tuberculous spondylitis from pyogenic spondylitis on MRI. AJR Am J Roentgenol 2004;182(6):1405–1410

Smith AS, Weinstein MA, Mizushima A, et al. MR imaging characteristics of tuberculous spondylitis vs vertebral osteomyelitis. AJR Am J Roentgenol 1989;153(2):399–405

## Case 80

Lai PH, Ho JT, Chen WL, et al. Brain abscess and necrotic brain tumor: discrimination with proton MR spectroscopy and diffusion-weighted imaging. AJNR Am J Neuroradiol 2002;23(8):1369–1377

Lai PH, Weng HH, Chen CY, et al. In vivo differentiation of aerobic brain abscesses and necrotic glioblastomas multiforme using proton MR spectroscopic imaging. AJNR Am J Neuroradiol 2008;29(8):1511–1518

Smirniotopoulos JG, Murphy FM, Rushing EJ, Rees JH, Schroeder JW. Patterns of contrast enhancement in the brain and meninges. Radiographics 2007;27(2):525–551

## Case 81

Biondi A, Jean B, Vivas E, et al. Giant and large peripheral cerebral aneurysms: etiopathologic considerations, endovascular treatment, and long-term follow-up. AJNR Am J Neuroradiol 2006;27(8):1685–1692

Chapot R, Houdart E, Saint-Maurice J-P, et al. Endovascular treatment of cerebral mycotic aneurysms. Radiology 2002;222(2):389–396

Kannoth S, Thomas SV, Nair S, Sarma PS. Proposed diagnostic criteria for intracranial infectious aneurysms. J Neurol Neurosurg Psychiatry 2008;79(8):943–946

## Case 82

Fujikawa A, Tsuchiya K, Honya K, Nitatori T. Comparison of MRI sequences to detect ventriculitis. AJR Am J Roentgenol 2006;187(4):1048–1053

Fukui MB, Williams RL, Mudigonda S. CT and MR imaging features of pyogenic ventriculitis. AJNR Am J Neuroradiol 2001;22(8):1510–1516

Pezzullo JA, Tung GA, Mudigonda S, Rogg JM, Diffusion-Weighted MR. Diffusion-weighted MR imaging of pyogenic ventriculitis. AJR Am J Roentgenol 2003;180(1):71–75

## Case 83

Rossi A. Imaging of acute disseminated encephalomyelitis. Neuroimaging Clin N Am 2008;18(1):149–161, ix

Young NP, Weinshenker BG, Lucchinetti CF. Acute disseminated encephalomyelitis: current understanding and controversies. Semin Neurol 2008;28(1):84–94

## Case 84

Ukisu R, Kushihashi T, Tanaka E, et al. Diffusion-weighted MR imaging of early-stage Creutzfeldt-Jakob disease: typical and atypical manifestations. Radiographics 2006;26(suppl 1):S191–S204

Wada R, Kucharczyk W. Prion infections of the brain. Neuroimaging Clin N Am 2008;18(1):183–191, ix

## Case 85

Ge Y. Multiple sclerosis: the role of MR imaging. AJNR Am J Neuroradiol 2006;27(6):1165–1176

Inglese M. Multiple sclerosis: new insights and trends. AJNR Am J Neuroradiol 2006;27(5):954–957

## Case 86

Thurnher MM, Cartes-Zumelzu F, Mueller-Mang C. Demyelinating and infectious diseases of the spinal cord. Neuroimaging Clin N Am 2007;17(1):37–55

## Case 87

Martin RJ. Central pontine and extrapontine myelinolysis: the osmotic demyelination syndromes. J Neurol Neurosurg Psychiatry 2004;75(suppl 3):iii22–iii28

Ruzek KA, Campeau NG, Miller GM. Early diagnosis of central pontine myelinolysis with diffusion-weighted imaging. AJNR Am J Neuroradiol 2004;25(2):210–213

## Case 88

Gallucci M, Limbucci N, Paonessa A, Splendiani A. Degenerative disease of the spine. Neuroimaging Clin N Am 2007;17(1):87–103

Modic MT, Ross JS. Lumbar degenerative disk disease. Radiology 2007;245(1):43–61

## Case 89

Gallucci M, Limbucci N, Paonessa A, Splendiani A. Degenerative disease of the spine. Neuroimaging Clin N Am 2007;17(1):87–103

## Case 90

Gebarski SS, Blaivas MA. Imaging of normal leptomeningeal melanin. AJNR Am J Neuroradiol 1996;17(1):55–60

Hsu WC, Loevner LA, Forman MS, Thaler ER. Superficial siderosis of the CNS associated with multiple cavernous malformations. AJNR Am J Neuroradiol 1999;20(7):1245–1248

Khalatbari K. Case 141: superficial siderosis. Radiology 2009;250(1):292–297

Uchino A, Aibe H, Itoh H, Aiko Y, Tanaka M. Superficial siderosis of the central nervous system. Its MRI manifestations. Clin Imaging 1997;21(4):241–245

## Case 91

Koenigsberg RA, Vakil N, Hong TA, et al. Evaluation of platybasia with MR imaging. AJNR Am J Neuroradiol 2005;26(1):89–92

Smoker WR. MR imaging of the craniovertebral junction. Magn Reson Imaging Clin N Am 2000;8(3):635–650

Smoker WR, Khanna G. Imaging the craniocervical junction. Childs Nerv Syst 2008;24(10):1123–1145

## Case 92

Abdelkarim A, Green R, Startzell J, Preece J. Craniofacial polyostotic fibrous dysplasia: a case report and review of the literature. Oral Surg Oral Med Oral Pathol Oral Radiol Endod 2008;106(1):e49–e55

Iseri PK, Efendi H, Demirci A, Komsuoglu S. Fibrous dysplasia of the cranial bones: a case report and review of the literature. Yale J Biol Med 2005;78(3):141–145

Tehranzadeh J, Fung Y, Donohue M, Anavim A, Pribram HW. Computed tomography of Paget disease of the skull versus fibrous dysplasia. Skeletal Radiol 1998;27(12):664–672

## Case 93

Ashley WW Jr, McKinstry RC, Leonard JR, Smyth MD, Lee BC, Park TS. Use of rapid-sequence magnetic resonance imaging for evaluation of hydrocephalus in children. J Neurosurg 2005; **103**(2 suppl)124–130

Lane JI, Luetmer PH, Atkinson JL. Corpus callosal signal changes in patients with obstructive hydrocephalus after ventriculoperitoneal shunting. AJNR Am J Neuroradiol 2001;22(1):158–162

Vertinsky AT, Barnes PD. Macrocephaly, increased intracranial pressure, and hydrocephalus in the infant and young child. Top Magn Reson Imaging 2007;18(1):31–51

## Case 94

Bradley WG. Normal pressure hydrocephalus: new concepts on etiology and diagnosis. AJNR Am J Neuroradiol 2000;21(9):1586–1590

Graff-Radford NR. Normal pressure hydrocephalus. Neurol Clin 2007;25(3):809–832, vii–viii

## Case 95

Bartynski WS. Posterior reversible encephalopathy syndrome, part 1: fundamental imaging and clinical features. AJNR Am J Neuroradiol 2008;29(6):1036–1042

Bartynski WS, Boardman JF. Distinct imaging patterns and lesion distribution in posterior reversible encephalopathy syndrome. AJNR Am J Neuroradiol 2007;28(7):1320–1327

## Case 96

Koyama T, Ueda H, Togashi K, Umeoka S, Kataoka M, Nagai S. Radiologic manifestations of sarcoidosis in various organs. Radiographics 2004;24(1):87–104

Lury KM, Smith JK, Matheus MG, Castillo M. Neurosarcoidosis—review of imaging findings. Semin Roentgenol 2004;39(4):495–504

## Case 97

Bote RP, Blázquez-Llorca L, Fernández-Gil MA, Alonso-Nanclares L, Muñoz A, De Felipe J. Hippocampal sclerosis: histopathology substrate and magnetic resonance imaging. Semin Ultrasound CT MR 2008;29(1):2–14

Deblaere K, Achten E. Structural magnetic resonance imaging in epilepsy. Eur Radiol 2008;18(1):119–129

Van Paesschen W. Qualitative and quantitative imaging of the hippocampus in mesial temporal lobe epilepsy with hippocampal sclerosis. Neuroimaging Clin N Am 2004;14(3):373–400, vii

## Case 98

Armao D, Castillo M, Chen H, Kwock L. Colloid cyst of the third ventricle: imaging-pathologic correlation. AJNR Am J Neuroradiol 2000;21(8):1470–1477

El Khoury C, Brugières P, Decq P, et al. Colloid cysts of the third ventricle: are MR imaging patterns predictive of difficulty with percutaneous treatment? AJNR Am J Neuroradiol 2000;21(3):489–492

## Case 99

Jacobs DA, Galetta SL. Neuro-ophthalmology for neuroradiologists. AJNR Am J Neuroradiol 2007;28(1):3–8

Jäger HR, Miszkiel KA. Pathology of the optic nerve. Neuroimaging Clin N Am 2008;18(2):243–259, x

## Case 100

Madoff DC, Wallace MJ, Ahrar K, Saxon RR. TIPS-related hepatic encephalopathy: management options with novel endovascular techniques. Radiographics 2004;24(1):21–36, discussion 36–37

Matsusue E, Kinoshita T, Ohama E, Ogawa T. Cerebral cortical and white matter lesions in chronic hepatic encephalopathy: MR-pathologic correlations. AJNR Am J Neuroradiol 2005;26(2):347–351

Mínguez B, Rovira A, Alonso J, Córdoba J. Decrease in the volume of white matter lesions with improvement of hepatic encephalopathy. AJNR Am J Neuroradiol 2007;28(8):1499–1500

Rovira A, Alonso J, Córdoba J. MR imaging findings in hepatic encephalopathy. AJNR Am J Neuroradiol 2008;29(9):1612–1621

# Index

Note: Locators are case numbers. **Boldface** numbers indicate discussion of primary diagnosis.